Praise for

The Cancer Survivor's Companion

"As Jenny's oncologist, I told her that it was a part of her treatment to get outside, keep moving and stay engaged with the world. Despite some challenges along the way, her outside garden activities have absolutely helped her to heal and find hope. *The Cancer Survivor's Garden Companion* will be a valuable resource for people at any stage of cancer treatment and recovery."

~ **Dr. Carlos Rubin de Celis,** Oncologist, Texas Oncology

"Jenny's beautiful book reminds us all that life can be found in the healing, meditative act of gardening. By lovingly tending a garden, we can learn to nurture ourselves, restoring our mind, body and spirit in the process."

~ **Ray Anne Evans,** Executive Director, Breast Cancer Resource Centers of Texas

"Jenny's connection with gardening, garden design, and simply being in nature remained strong throughout her cancer diagnosis, treatment, and recovery. In fact, it was part of what helped her through. And now she is helping others to learn from her powerful experience.

"In this book, Jenny's personality lights up each page with her intelligence, honesty, hopefulness and wit. Gardeners struggling with cancer will feel as if a good friend is there beside them, encouraging them to keep doing what they love to do. Non-gardeners may want to start! Friends and family will also benefit, understanding their loved one's experience in a new light and, perhaps, being inspired to connect with them in the garden."

~ **Naomi A. Sachs,** Founding Director, Therapeutic Landscapes Network;
co-author, *Therapeutic Landscapes: An Evidence-Based Approach to Designing Healing Gardens and Restorative Outdoor Spaces*

"Jenny's tips for incorporating gardening into your life for mind, body, and spiritual health are ingenious! As a cancer coach, I will definitely be suggesting this book to my clients."

~ **Susan Gonzalez, BSN, CPCC,**
co-author of *100 Perks of Having Cancer Plus 100 Health Tips for Surviving It,*
and editor of The Savvy Sister blog

"*The Cancer Survivor's Garden Companion* is an inspiring guide to the spiritual journey awaiting you in your own backyard. As a cancer survivor and garden designer, Jenny Peterson writes with authority, positive energy and an understanding heart. What she discovered in her personal journey will galvanize any cancer survivor who is open to possibilities to see the garden as a tool for healing and well-being. A beautiful, informative, and wise book."

~ **Fran Sorin,** author of *Digging Deep: Unearthing Your Creative Roots Through Gardening,*
10th Anniversary Edition

"Jenny Peterson has eloquently and candidly put into words perhaps the most important and powerful reason for gardens – their therapeutic power to heal mind and body."

~ **Joe Lamp'l,** Executive Producer and Host of "Growing a Greener World"

"Get this book! Whether you are a gardener, a cancer patient or survivor, or caretaking someone who is, you need to read this book. As a doctor and gardener myself, I can assure you her approach is spot on; not only will your garden soothe your spirit, it can literally heal your body. Seeing your garden as a reflection of your own physical, mental, spiritual and emotional bodies can provide a fabulous mirror for self-healing. I preach the benefits of being grounded to my patients; there's no better way than gardening and this book will lead you there."

~ **Dr. Robin Mayfield,** DC, A.C.N., featured in *Five Steps to Selecting the Best Alternative Medicine*

"Jenny Peterson is an inspiration to all who know her and the best friend you can have. Her message of overcoming the fear of a frightening disease by finding peace and purpose in the garden is one that will resonate with anyone whose life has been touched by cancer."

~ **Steve Bender,** Senior Garden Writer, *Southern Living* magazine

"Jenny's engaging, heartwarming and down-to-earth style of writing is like having a best friend by your side as you navigate through this 'interruption' in your daily life. Jenny's advice is spot-on, and I only wish this book was available when I was diagnosed with cancer. As Jenny says, 'You're a gardener, and gardeners believe in possibilities.' Truer words were never spoken!"

~ **Rebecca Sweet,** garden designer and author of
Refresh Your Garden Design with Color, Texture and Form

"Jenny Peterson reminds us that we are more than a job or a diagnosis. We are spiritual beings held together by a larger creative force – and we can see evidence of this in the gardens we plan and tend. A great manual for life living."

~ Andie Redwine, filmmaker, "Paradise Recovered"

"As a psychologist/horticultural therapist, I have great faith in the healing power of gardening, which played a critical role in my personal recovery from stage 3 cancer. In *The Cancer Survivor's Garden Companion,* Jenny Peterson guides you to view your garden as an invaluable resource in your healing journey. This book shows that gardening is more than an act of faith for cancer survivors, it is also an act of self-love and of healing."

~ Florence Strang, M.Ed., co-author of *100 Perks of Having Cancer Plus 100 Health Tips for Surviving It*

"Jenny Peterson chose the perfect title for this book: *The Cancer Survivor's Garden Companion: Cultivating Hope, Healing and Joy in the Ground Beneath Your Feet.* Jenny sees the garden as a field where health, hope and joy can spring from – but more importantly, where nature offers a healing companionship. How so?

"Facing a cancer diagnosis, Jenny has the perfect excuse to abandon her garden and focus on tending to her own needs. Instead, she turns to the garden as a physical and emotional outlet. And she reaps spiritual comfort from her gardening tasks. Jenny's beautiful book offers practical suggestions for nurturing a win/win relationship with nature during challenging times. This isn't a 'pie in the sky' philosophy, it's a down to earth approach for standing tall while digging in!"

~ Shirley Bovshow, Eden-maker and landscape designer; garden design expert on the Hallmark Channel's "Home and Family" show.

" *The Cancer Survivor's Garden Companion* brilliantly illustrates the ways people and plants can be healers of themselves and others in a purposeful community-driven environment."

~ LaManda Joy, Founder and Executive Director, Chicago's Peterson Garden Project, board member of the American Community Gardening Association

"Jenny Peterson shows how gardening properly and safely can not only help you feel better, it can help your body strengthen and heal from cancer treatment and its after-effects. This is a great resource for every cancer survivor!"

~ Jacqueline Jensen, CLT, Doctor of Physical Therapy

"With spunk, humor and spiritual sensitivity, Jenny Peterson takes us down the scary road of cancer to find our true sense of self. Her journey to essential awareness transcends all struggles, regardless of origin."

~ **Linda Lehmusvirta,** Producer, PBS's "Central Texas Gardener"

"On the days in your recovery when you can't imagine getting out of bed, much less working in the garden, Jenny's friendly tone and concrete suggestions for how to begin -- no matter how slowly -- will inspire and motivate you. Moreover, the story of how Jenny used her love of gardening as a tool in her own recovery struck a chord in me, as it will surely do for you."

~ **Denise Mickelsen,** Gardening Acquisitions Editor, Craftsy

"Having cancer affects life in ways that people who have never experienced it could never imagine. In *The Cancer Survivor's Garden Companion*, Jenny Peterson draws on her love of gardening and shares how it inspired her and helped carry her through her own challenging experience with the disease. Brutally honest at times, and endearing at others, no one tells it like it is the way Jenny does, and offers solutions and celebrations that not only help those dealing with cancer, but also anyone who has ever felt overwhelmed with life. This book is 192 pages filled with hope and encouragement."

~ **Kylee Baumle,** co-author of *Indoor Plant Décor,* book review editor for *Horticulture* magazine

"Jenny writes from the heart, with hard-won knowledge, about living with and surviving cancer – all with the help of her beloved garden, which during her treatment and recovery offered daily moments of beauty and spiritual and emotional healing. 'Allow your garden to bring you joy,' she advises fellow gardeners living with cancer. In this hopeful yet practical guide, she shows how a garden can soothe and heal."

~ **Pam Penick,** landscape designer and author of *Lawn Gone!*

"At the best of times, a garden is a place of joy, action and energy; in times of stress, it can be a haven of peace, solace and perspective. In her book, Jenny Peterson skillfully weaves first-hand experience with practical advice on engaging with a garden for mental, spiritual and physical renewal – as a way to cope with the process of diagnosis, treatment and recovery. Her gentle, encouraging style will surely be a gift to seasoned gardeners struggling with limited time and energy, as well as not-yet-gardeners looking for a way to connect with the healing power of the outdoors."

~ **Nancy J. Ondra,** garden writer, author of *Five Plant Gardens*

The

Cancer Survivor's
Garden Companion

The

Cancer Survivor's
Garden Companion

CULTIVATING HOPE, HEALING AND JOY IN THE GROUND BENEATH YOUR FEET

Jenny Peterson

st. lynn's
press

PITTSBURGH

The Cancer Survivor's Garden Companion
Cultivating Hope, Healing and Joy in the Ground Beneath Your Feet

ISBN-13: 978-0-9892688-9-9

Library of Congress Control Number: 2015947990
CIP information available upon request

First Edition, 2016

St. Lynn's Press • POB 18680 • Pittsburgh, PA 15236
412.381.9933 • www.stlynnspress.com

Book design – Holly Rosborough
Editor – Catherine Dees

Photo credits:
All photos are by Jenny Peterson except for the following:
Brett Davis – xviii, xx, 12, 22, 25, 26, 29, 76, 83, 158-159, 169; Bill Bastas – 2, 3, 4 (left), 5 (top), 7, 8, 11, 32, 94, 97, 108; Kylee Baumle – xii; Tom Urban – 78, 85; Michael Urban – 86, 87-88, 89, 90-91; Bonnie Plants – 35, 48, 50, 52, 53 (all), 57, 62 (top), 166, 171; Ruby Cortez – 4 (right); Beth Bizer - 23; Christy Ten Eyck – 36, 44; Naomi Sachs – 42 (top left); Linda Lehmusvirta – 101; Patti Waldrup – 103; Michael Moreno – 138; Lisa Jennings - 147 (bottom left); Michael Paolini – 157 (top); Shawna Coronado – 160; Holly Rosborough – across from Table of Contents, 66 (bottom left), 74 (top right), 106, 111, 112 (bottom left), 151, 171
Graphic Background Embellishments: Design by www.123Freevectors.com

DISCLAIMER

The author and publisher expressly disclaim any responsibility for any adverse effects occurring as a result of the suggestions or information herein. The information in this book is based on the author's personal thoughts and experience, and is not intended to be a substitute for the medical advice of a licensed, trained physician or health professional. For all medical questions, the reader should consult the appropriate health care practitioners.

Printed in China
On certified FSC recycled paper using soy-based inks

This title and all of St. Lynn's Press books may be purchased for educational,
business or sales promotional use. For information please write:
Special Markets Department . St. Lynn's Press . POB 18680 . Pittsburgh, PA 15236

10 9 8 7 6 5 4 3 2 1

Dedicated with great love in memory of my parents

Richard Nybro
(1925-1999, liver cancer)

and

Jennie Andreasen Nybro
(1929-1989, breast cancer)

*who taught us all how to live with grace and joy
regardless of circumstance.*

And in profound gratitude for my children

Maxwell and Luke

*who teach me daily how to live
with humor and a sense of possibility.*

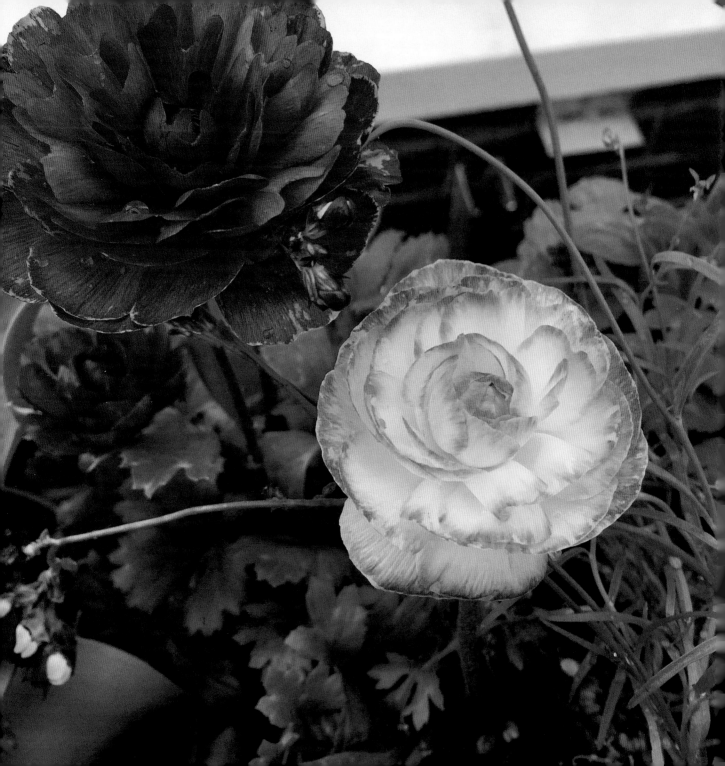

Table of Contents

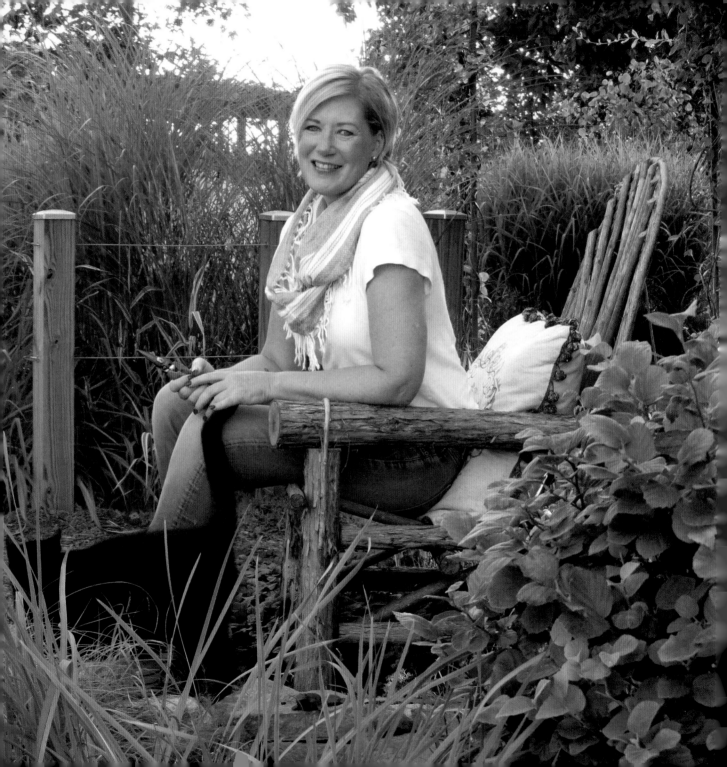

The Garden That Heals

"Don't let cancer define you, Jenny. You are more than your diagnosis."

This was the advice from my doctor when she gave me the news that I had breast cancer, the disease that had killed my mother. It was Friday, May 11, 2012 – I don't need to look up the date because it's seared into my memory, like it is for most people with a cancer diagnosis. I thought, "That's easy for you to say. You don't have breast cancer."

Then I met my oncologist, who said, "Not everything in your world can be about breast cancer." So clearly I had a theme going here, and it made me think beyond my feelings of fear and panic. Who am I, aside from being a person with breast cancer? Who was I before this diagnosis, and had she changed?

The answer is that I am many things. I am Jenny. I am a gardener. I am a writer. I am a mother. I am a fiancée, a sister, a friend. I am a designer. I am a child of God. I am optimistic, sarcastically funny, and I am a good baker. There's no reason I can't still be all of those things even after my diagnosis, right?

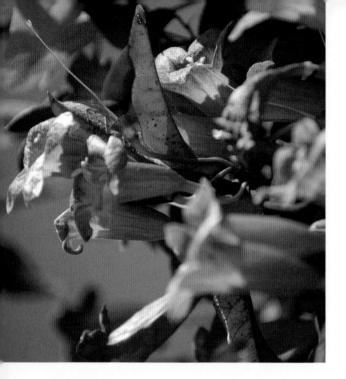

Yet I struggled with my feelings of competency, I questioned my physical and mental abilities, and I yearned for the days when the world around me felt secure and recognizable. If you've had a cancer diagnosis, you've probably felt the same. Your world has changed forever, and you don't know how you'll navigate all of the changes. Your body doesn't move and feel the same, and it certainly doesn't look the same if you've had any amount of surgery. You may question your attractiveness and your vitality, your inner and outer strength.

"Don't let cancer define you, Jenny."

So how did I not let cancer define me? Not knowing anything better, I simply kept doing what I knew to do. And one of those things was gardening. Plants, and the act of growing and caring for them, have been a central part of my personal and professional life for a long time. I'm a freelance garden writer and author as well as a garden designer, and I've gardened on a 150-square-foot garden as well as an entire acre. I love houseplants, flowers, succulents and herbs. So I gardened.

For a long time, my gardening didn't resemble the type of gardening I used to do. I was weak, and struggled with some range of motion issues in my left arm where I'd had surgery. I felt a little depressed and lacked energy, and I was sensitive to heat. I was told to not lift more than 10 pounds and to not perform repetitive, jarring motions. That kind of left out shoveling, wheelbarrowing and plant hauling. What to do, what to do.

I'm not going to lie – I had many days when I did not feel like gardening. But I decided to change my approach and focus on small, doable tasks. I could water my front porch plants and tend to

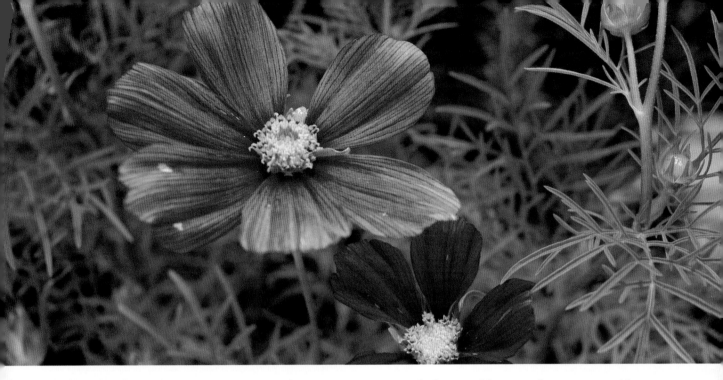

my houseplants without any problem, so that's what I did most days. And little by little, my relationship with plants and my garden became the thing that turned me around – body, mind and spirit. No, it wasn't easy. Nothing about cancer and cancer treatment is easy. But it was my reality, and I was determined to find some place where I could thrive and experience joy again.

And you will, too. This book is not a how-to, because everybody's journey is different. I wrote this book as a way of helping you find a way to enjoy your life and the world around you, even if you have cancer. If you have this book in your hands, you are a gardener or you want to be one. Your garden – no matter how large or small, how grand or humble – can be a place of beauty and refuge for you at a time when you need it the most. It can help to strengthen you and widen your world, and it can remind you of who you are. Your garden can be a garden that heals...a companion on your journey.

So don't let cancer define you. You're a gardener, and gardeners believe in possibilities. ❧

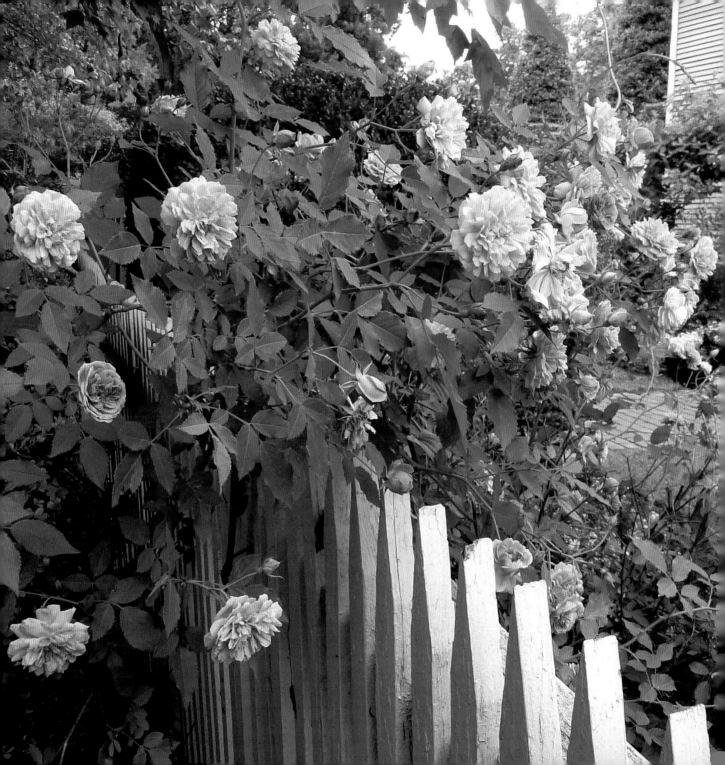

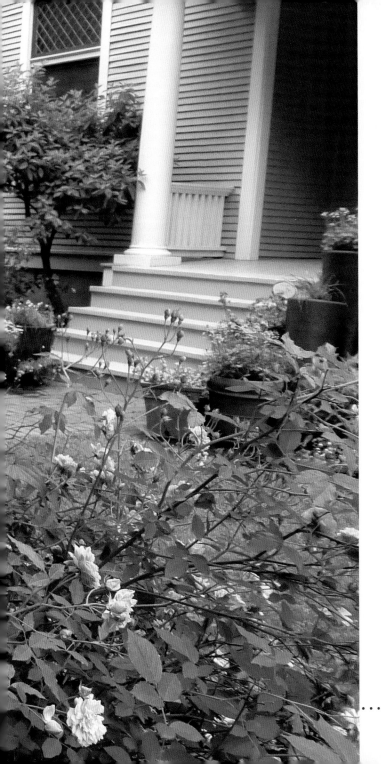

What's Inside

*B*efore we get started, I want to talk with you about what is in this book exactly, and what you can expect from it. It's not a gardening "how-to" manual – there are many books out there that tell you exactly how to plant something, how to treat oak wilt and how to sow seeds. This is not that book. This book is to encourage people who are diagnosed with cancer, going through cancer treatment, healing from cancer or living with cancer to view their gardens, plants and outdoor spaces as resources in creating the healthiest and most balanced life possible. Life can be difficult, but it can also be profoundly beautiful, and our gardens are the best teachers of this.

This book has three sections: **Body**, **Mind** and **Spirit**. Many people (myself included) have a tendency to confuse Mind and Spirit, so I thought it would be helpful to give my definitions.

BODY: Our physical being is described as our Body. Brains, cells, muscles, blood, senses, tendons, hormones, nerves,

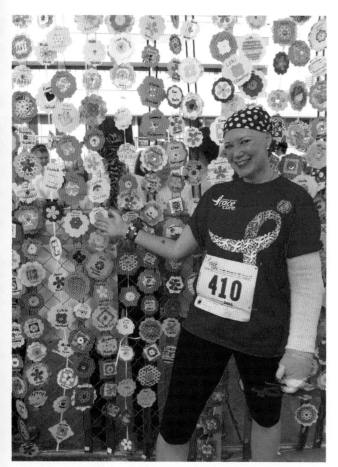

bones – everything physical about us is contained in a body, and that's what this section is about. Our physical sensations can affect our minds and vice-versa, but they are not the same.

MIND: Our minds deal with emotions, will, decisions, feelings, choices, moods, even rational intellect. Everything we think and feel comes from our minds – our perceptions of reality, how we understand ourselves, how we relate to others and descriptions of our own personalities...all reside in the Mind.

SPIRIT: Many people think of your "spirit" as describing your emotions and mood. Emotions and mood are actually a part of one's Mind, at least for my working definition for this book. Your Spirit deals with issues of meaning, essence, faith, energy, "God," Universe, purpose, spirituality and "Higher Power." You don't need to be religious or even believe in God or a Higher Power to gain use from this section. Use the Spirit section to connect with the deepest part of who you are, however it is you define that. I will use different terms from various teachings, but feel free to insert your own.

Although my own experience has been with skin cancer and breast cancer, this book is for people who have experienced all forms of cancer, for people of any age, for men and women alike, and for new gardeners and experienced ones. Cancer does not discriminate, and I don't, either.

Throughout this book you will see images of people performing all kinds of garden activities. All of these people are cancer survivors; no models were used. You'll also see boxes with what I call "Survivor Spotlights" – these are quick views into the lives of gardeners who are cancer survivors, and you can see what their diagnoses were and read their tips for getting through diagnosis and treatment. Gardeners are the best people to share everything – divisions, cuttings, coffee and cancer advice.

You'll notice that I have included a few screenshots of text messages and Facebook posts randomly throughout the book. These messages and comments between my family, friends and me (and sometimes strangers on Facebook) served as a kind of journal to me throughout my diagnosis and treatment. When I look back on them and read them with new, fresh eyes, it is very moving to me that I had the love and well wishes of so many people.

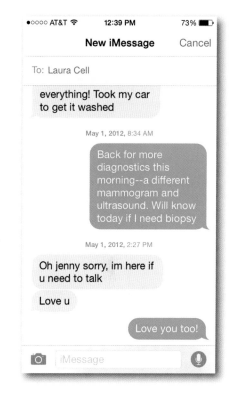

When I feel discouraged about my recovery from time to time, I can simply go back and read these messages of support, encouragement and incredible love – they remind me that my Tribe is so much bigger than I ever dreamed it could be. I hope that they can remind you of how large your Tribe is.

You'll also notice that I often stress talking with your doctor before doing anything in this book. Whether we are talking about an oncologist, a surgeon, a holistic doctor, a rehab therapist – whoever it is that helps you manage your treatment and care – those people need to be consulted first before you make

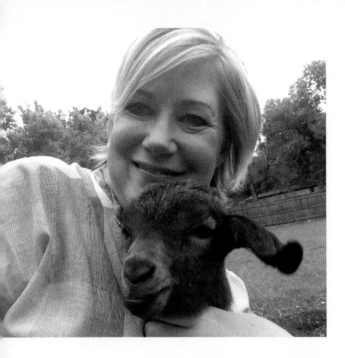

a Master's degree in Theology, and I'm a writer and a landscaper. Some would say I collected oddball degrees and certifications along the way, and I can't say that I disagree with them. I never imagined how all of the education I've received and my life experiences would come together in one book, but that is exactly what has happened. Call it serendipity if you will, but although I wouldn't go as far as to say that I am thankful for my breast cancer diagnosis, I can surely say that I am thankful for where it has led me. My life is forever changed, as I'm sure yours has been, by this diagnosis – but it's the combination of so many twists and turns in this life that have brought me to this point.

And I'm glad to meet you here. ⤳

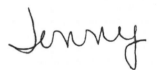

any changes to your treatment plan. It's impossible to overstress this point. I have a number of professionals at my disposal, and I rely on them to help me heal, and it's to my advantage to include them and consult them at every turn. So please, don't be a Lone Ranger here. I am not a physician, a therapist or a surgeon.

That brings me to my last point. I could never have guessed where my life would lead me, but I feel that it has led me directly to writing this book. I have a Bachelor's degree in Psychology,

body

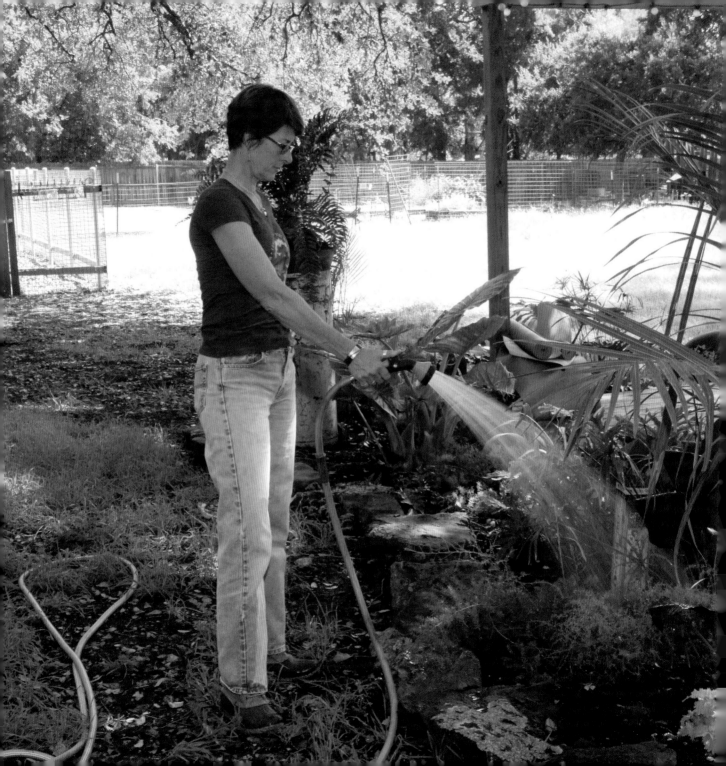

ONE

Sweat It Out

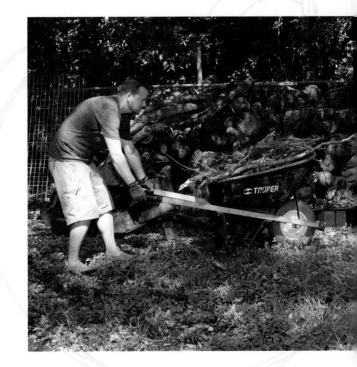

*E*xercise is good for everyone, but especially those going through treatment or healing from it. Caution is the word, however, as your body might not be able to do the things it once could. Take it slow and honor what your body has gone through and is going through, and let your garden help your body get stronger.

Surgery and treatment, whether it's chemotherapy or radiation, can really zap your immune system and physical energy. When I was going through treatment, my oncologist, Dr. Rubin de Celis, told me, "Consider it a part of your treatment to get regular exercise."

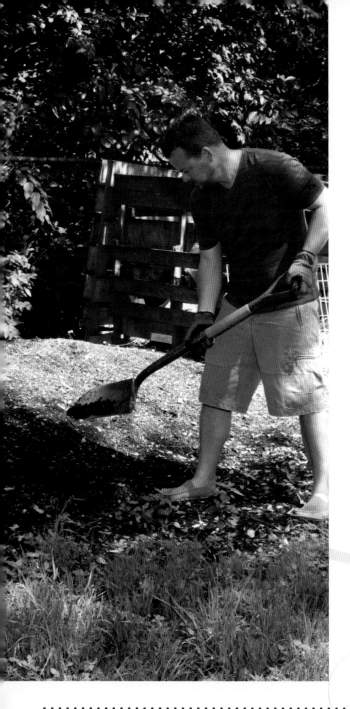

Cardio

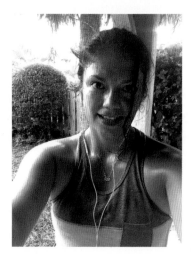

Given your doctor's approval, you can partici-pate in cardio exercises that will, over time, increase your stamina – but go slow and build up to longer sessions in the garden with greater intensity. This is particularly true for those who have lymphedema like I do, as the swelling in your limbs or torso can be greatly exacerbated by sudden changes in your physical exertion.

Some great garden chores for light cardio include:

- Hauling mulch bags, one at a time to start
- Turning your compost pile
- Shoveling compost into new beds
- Pushing a ½ full wheelbarrow up an incline
- Mowing your lawn
- Hoeing weeds

Safety First!

- Sunblock
- Wide-brimmed garden hat
- Compression garments, if necessary: glove, gauntlet, sleeve, bra, or trunk garment
- Bug repellent
- Sturdy shoes
- Gloves
- Surgical gloves to layer underneath garden gloves

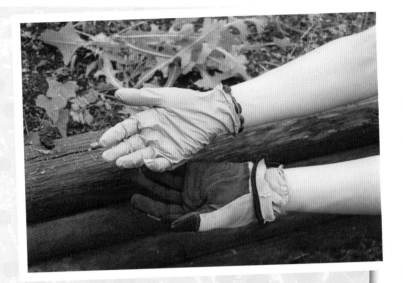

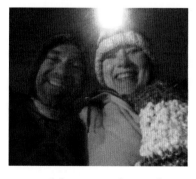

There was a time during my treatment, as the weather was getting colder, that we'd bought some winter vegetable transplants from the garden center. Those poor plants sat on our back patio for a couple of weeks because, frankly, I was exhausted and so was Brett, my fiancé. One day he texted me that we should get those plants in the ground.

I wish I still had those texts – we text so much that our carrier eventually deleted old messages to make room for new ones – but the conversation went something like this:

Brett: *On the way home; let's get those plants in the ground.*

Me: *But you'll be home late and it's cold outside.*

Brett: *Then get bundled up!*

Me: *But, it'll be dark!*

Brett: *I've got headlamps.*

Me: *Are you kidding me?*

Brett: *No way, Cupcake. Get a move on!*

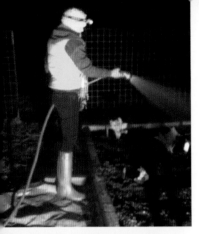

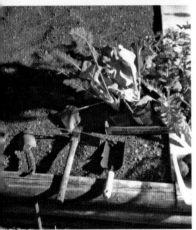

Now, I'm sure Brett really did want to get those transplants in the ground, but if we didn't and they died, we'd have only lost about $25. But more than that, I think he recognized that I hadn't been out to the garden in a while and he wanted me to be moving and active. Wise man.

So, forgive the terrible night shots on my old iPhone, but here is what we did and what I looked like! I had a cap on my bald head with a head-lamp over that, a hoodie with a puffy vest over it, my rubber rain boots, garden gloves and a scarf. Not a real fashion statement, but we got those transplants in the ground, watered them in, and laughed the entire time – it was good for our garden and even better for my soul.

Stretching and Flexibility

When you've had surgery and treatment, perhaps even ongoing treatment depending upon your stage, your body has undoubtedly been through a lot and it's got the kinks to show for it. I had a lymph node dissection after my sentinel lymph node came back unclear, and this surgery far surpassed my lumpectomy in every way possible. And I mean, "not in a good way." My nerves and muscles were severed underneath my left arm in order to get all the lymph nodes my surgeon could get his hands on. I'm not complaining, just stating the obvious – that kind of surgery is rough and has lasting effects! I have a lot of scar tissue all around my left underarm, and it constantly wants to pull my arm in and down.

So, the plan is to keep stretching it out. One way I do this is through yoga, and I also attend weekly rehab. But there are a number of garden activities that, when performed correctly, provide great stretching opportunities for your scar tissue and kinked-up muscles, increasing your range of motion and flexibility.

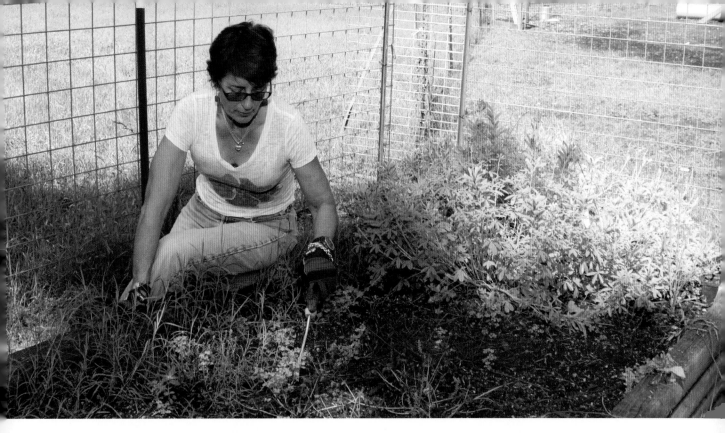

- Rake leaves and reach out just a bit farther than you think you might be able to.
- Hoe weeds, being careful if you have lymphedema.
- Shovel compost or soil.
- Hand weed, stretching across the bed or a little farther out from your body.
- Sit on the edge of your raised beds and stretch to the middle to maintain them.

- Avoid twisting your spine.
- Work with small instead of heavy loads.
- When lifting and carrying, keep objects close to your body.
- With stretching activities, you want to feel a nice stretch, not pain. If you experience pain, back off.
- Stay hydrated.

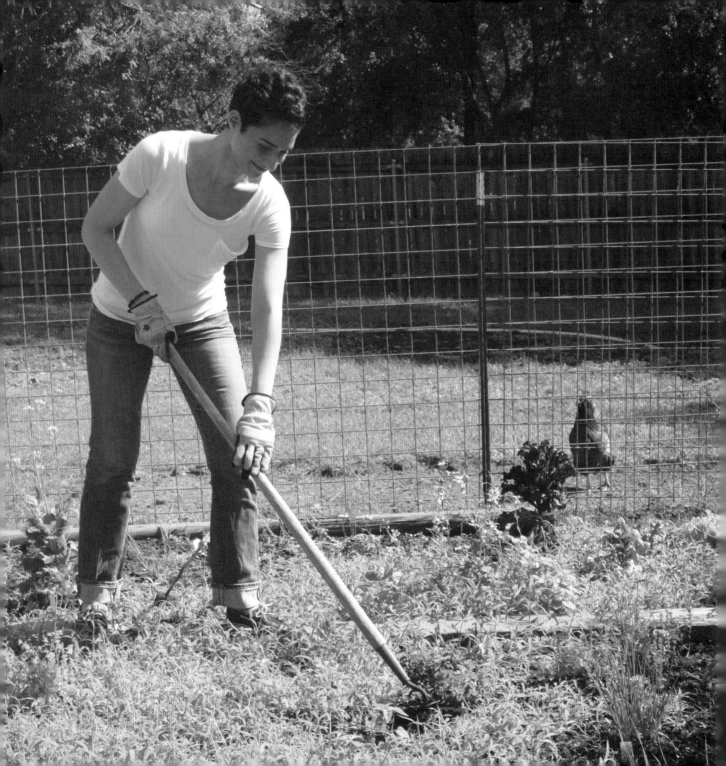

Strong Bones

Cancer doesn't care how old you are. I know many people who were diagnosed in their 20s and 30s as well as in their 50s and 60s (and beyond). So it may seem odd that a young person might need to think about keeping their bones strong, because we associate weak bones with age, don't we? But unfortunately, cancer patients who have had chemotherapy, steroid medications or hormone therapy can suffer from osteoporosis, or thinning of the bones. There are many things you can do to increase your bone strength – avoid tobacco products, limit alcohol, eat foods high in Vitamin D and calcium (hello, spinach, kale and okra!), and get regular exercise. Are you seeing your garden here?

Most any weight-bearing exercise will increase your bone strength, which is always a good thing, but particularly if you've gone through cancer treatment. Garden chores provide great opportunities for building bones, and while they may seem like they are the same types of activities as those I suggested for cardio (there is some overlap), the name of the game here is "slow and steady." And, as always, if you have recently had surgery or have any other limitation, do check with your doctor about appropriate and safe weight limits for lifting or carrying.

- Moving large pots or containers — be sure they are empty, though.
- Rearranging your patio furniture.
- Hauling one mulch bag at a time (think "pack mule," this isn't a race).
- Light wheelbarrowing on level ground.
- Turning the compost pile.
- Dragging tree limbs for disposal (not too heavy, though!).
- Dragging the hose around the garden (a 50' water-filled hose can be heavy).
- Unloading a 5-gallon plant from the back of your car.

Yoga

The benefits of yoga are numerous – increased flexibility, balance, circulation, positive lymphatic flow and mood enhancing – but how about yoga outside? We've all seen people in parks participating in public yoga, so consider bringing that same concept to your own backyard. Practicing yoga in the fresh air in the beauty of your own garden (or on your patio, deck or lawn) adds another layer of healing to this already restorative activity.

If you've practiced yoga before, you know there are many different types.

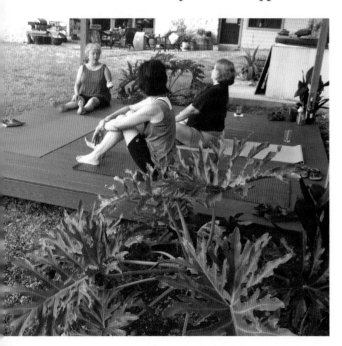

I used to do some very powerful yoga before my diagnosis, and then because I developed lymphedema, I had to reconsider my yoga practice. With the help of Rhonda, one of my lymphedema rehab therapists, I started with a very gentle type of yoga called "Restorative." I practiced that type for a number of months before slowly getting into more challenging poses. I'm still not where I was before, but I'm okay with it. If you are starting or restarting your yoga practice, here's a rundown of some of the more popular types of yoga and how they may or may not be what you need:

RESTORATIVE: Restorative yoga does not resemble the type of yoga most of us picture in our heads – the poses are almost all lying down, and your body is supported with blocks and straps so you can hold positions for a number of minutes. It's perfect for people going through treatment, recovery, or simply needing a healing session to induce calm and peace. It can also include chanting or gongs if you attend a class, but in your own practice, it's simply relaxing.

BIKRAM: This is "hot" yoga, where the studio is heated to 105 degrees F, with

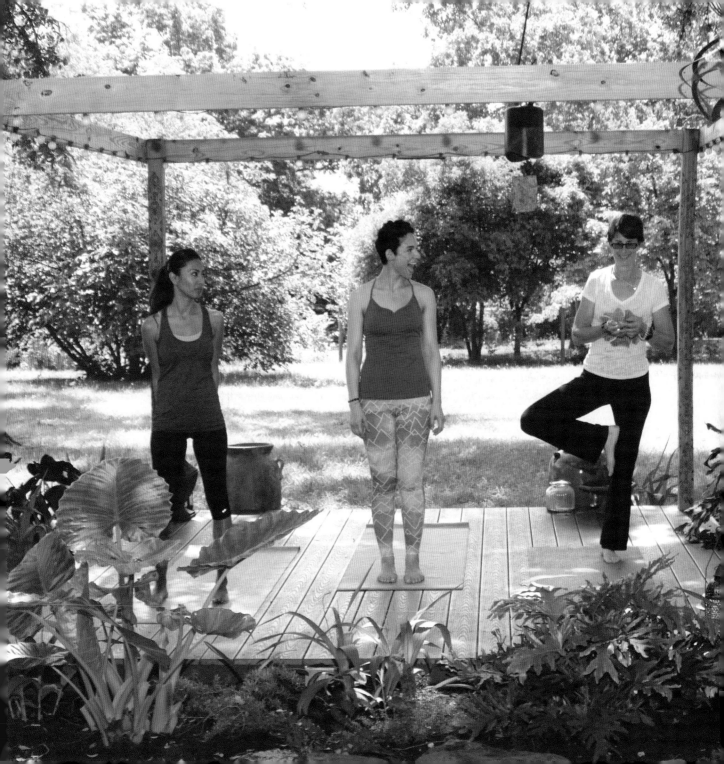

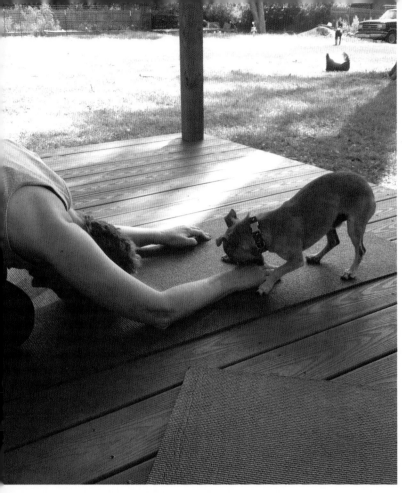

KUNDALINI: A gentler form of yoga, Kundalini yoga is 50 percent exercise, 20 percent breath work, 20 percent meditation, and 10 percent relaxation. It typically includes chanting, so if you are uncomfortable with this, you might want to choose a different type of yoga, but it's a great one for those going through or recovery from treatment.

HATHA: Ideal for beginners, Hatha yoga refers to any practice that combines poses with breathing techniques. Do it at your own pace to increase flexibility and balance and to induce calm.

VINYASA: This is a fairly fast-paced yoga, often called "power yoga," that requires constant movement through a flowing series of lunging, stretching and bending. You can work up to this type of yoga, but it is not recommended for those who have recently had surgery or treatment.

40% humidity. The heat loosens your muscles and increases your ability to stretch. It's comprised of a series of 26 poses completed twice, sandwiched in between breath work. Check with your doctor or rehab therapist first – those with lymphedema should avoid this, as heat exacerbates the associated swelling.

ASHTANGA: Ashtanga is a physically challenging yoga for seasoned practitioners, using up to 70 poses including back bends, inversion poses and sun salutations. This will most likely not be recommended initially, but it is definitely a type of yoga that you can work up to over a longer period of time.

My advice is to always check with your doctor or rehab therapist first (are you getting tired of hearing me say that yet?), start slow even though you may be experienced, and drop your expectation of doing a perfect Crane pose. Don't even make me laugh – I am so far away from Crane that it's kind of ridiculous. I may never do the Crane pose because it's a lot of weight on your arms, but it's possible I can work my way up to it. In the beginning, experiment with the standing and sitting poses as well as the ones that are performed lying down, as your balance may be a bit off for a while.

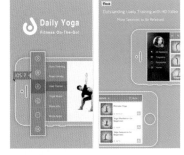

If you have an iPad or similar tablet, look up some apps for yoga to help you with your practice. I use one called "Daily Yoga" that has been my guide for about two years now. It offers different levels and lengths of sessions, and I started using it specifically because it included sessions using

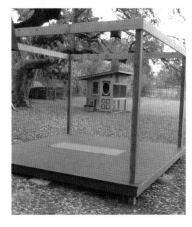

only seated or standing poses.

When I finished treatment, I was just shy of my 50th birthday. My fiancé is a "doer" and really wanted to give me something that would be useful to me as I healed. I had balance issues created by nerve damage in my feet from chemotherapy, I had scar tissue that continually wanted to pull my left arm down, my left side was weaker than my right, and I was fighting the Mood Rollercoaster. I also love to practice yoga. So, while I was gone for a week at a flower and garden show, Brett got to work with our carpenter friend, Jim, and built me a yoga deck.

I'd showed him pictures of similar decks before, but always followed with, "Wouldn't that be cool if..." What a lucky woman I am that I have a mate who took my words to heart! I returned from the trip to find a newly built yoga deck adjacent to our chicken coop.

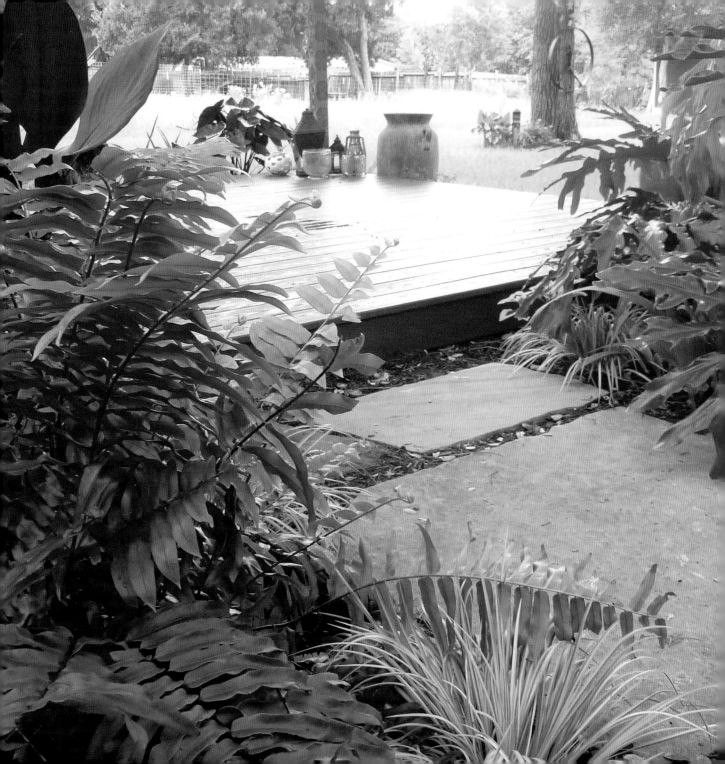

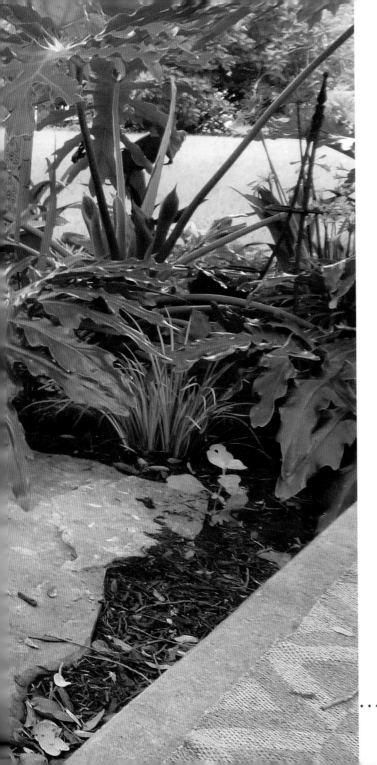

Many things have changed in the backyard since that deck was built – we built a huge chicken run around the coop, and created a tropical garden around the yoga deck. Now, it's still a very young garden, so the plants aren't yet as mature as I envision them to be, but what a gift to go out to that deck in the mornings with my coffee to practice yoga as the sun is just rising! And I may or may not practice at the end of the day with a beer; I will never tell.

It's a 12' x 12' square, so just large enough for about 4 people to practice yoga together, but perfect for solo practice as well. If you want to build a deck similar to this one, here are my recommendations:

Use a composite decking material such as Trex. It has a natural wood grain and comes in a variety of colors or "stains," and it can cost twice as much as real wood but you never have to maintain it. I like it because there is zero risk of getting splinters in your feet or hands – very important if you have lymphedema in your leg or arm and are susceptible to infections like I am!

Make it just a little larger than you think you'll need, 10' x 10' minimum.

Some yoga poses are challenging, and combined with my balance issues, I fall over frequently. Better to fall on a deck than off of one.

Have some kind of lighting at or around your deck. I sometimes like to go out very early in the morning or even late at night when the light is dim, and the last thing I want to do is trip because I can't see where I'm going. If lighting doesn't fit within your budget, bring a flashlight.

Install a waist-high bar for balance poses – we've talked about doing this with my yoga deck but haven't gotten around to it yet. It's nice to know that you can quickly hold onto something if you feel yourself going down.

Plant choices for a yoga deck garden

As I created the garden around my deck, I really wanted to have a sense of calm, peace and tranquility, so I chose plants that are tropical in nature, lush, soft and colorful. While I love agaves (and they make sense in my Texas garden) I wouldn't dream of planting anything spiky or pokey here. Consider some of these plants:

Ornamental Grasses:
Miscanthus spp.
Pennisetum spp.
Festuca spp.

Big-leafed tropicals:
Colocasia spp.
Canna spp.
Philodendron spp.

Exotic foliage:
Coleus spp.
Calathea spp.
Anthurium spp.
Croton spp.

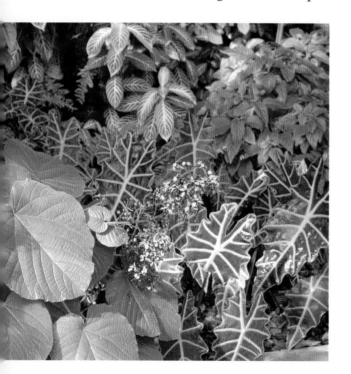

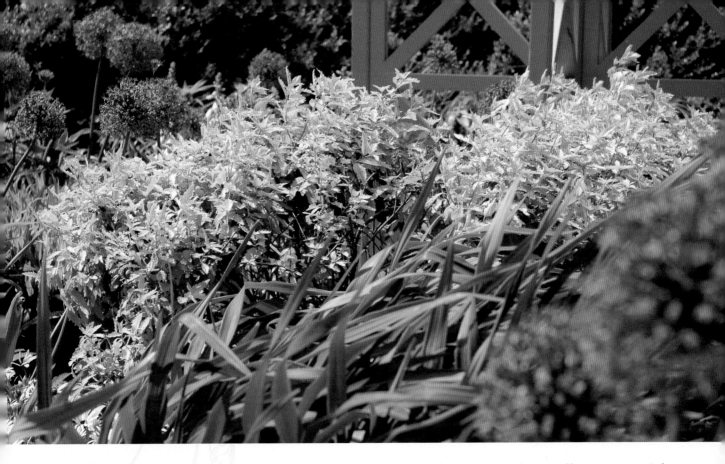

The ferns:
Adiantum spp.
Nephrolepis spp.
Platycerium spp.
Asplenium spp.

Bamboo is also a great choice as it's a very "zen" plant, but be sure you are choosing the clumping variety rather than the spreading kind, which can quickly overtake your yard as well as your neighbor's. Believe me, planting spreading bamboo will quickly use up any cancer sympathy you have from your neighbors. Even if they don't say anything, they will give you the Stink Eye forevermore.

I want to stress that my yoga deck garden is the only garden I really tend on our property. It's the one that is the most important to me, the one that is the most

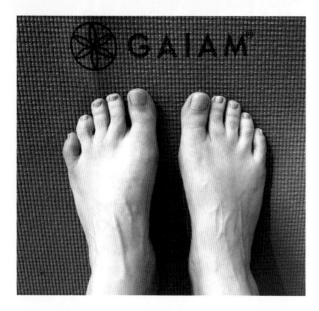

post-diagnosis, and while my body, mind and spirit have healed dramatically during that time, I am still aware of my limits and boundaries. It's good to push them so I continue to move forward with my healing. This garden has proven to be the balm that helps to make me whole again.

And remember – there is a reason why yoga is called a "practice." This is not about being perfect and judging yourself. Even the healthiest of bodies fluctuate day-to-day in terms of flexibility and strength, so the goal here is to honor where your body is at this very moment, and let your garden help move it forward. ⌒

life-giving and healing to me, and the one that I can realistically keep up with. At the writing of this book, I'm three years

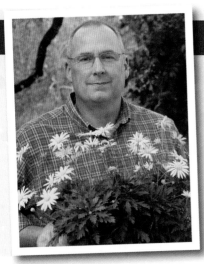

Survivor Spotlight

Name: Rick

Age at diagnosis: 29

Diagnosis: Testicular Cancer (Embryonal Cell Carcinoma)

Stage: 3–A

Tip: Let your garden be what you need it to be on any given day. Sometimes, a quiet retreat where you can contemplate and focus. Other times, a place to just get lost in gardening and take your mind off of things.

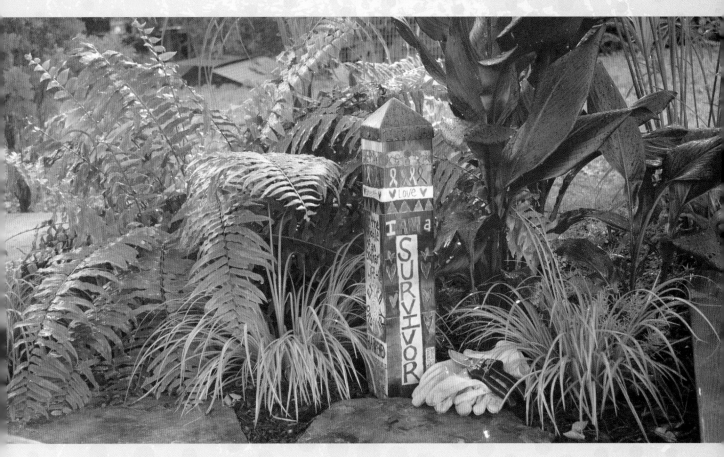

The Christmas after I finished treatment, my friends Sherry and Jacque gave me this Survivor peace pole, which has a place of honor in my garden. It reminds me every day I see it to live with hope and joy. My peace pole was designed by artist Stephanie Burgess, who is a breast cancer survivor. It includes messages of hope and encouragement on each of the four sides, and features cancer awareness ribbons of each color around the top. It nestles happily among the plants in my yoga deck garden, and although it looks larger in the photo, it is only 20 inches high and 4 inches square. Stephanie's work can be found online: Painted Peace-Wood Art of Stephanie Joan Burgess-Peace Poles, Planks and Wall Art (www.paintedpeace.com).

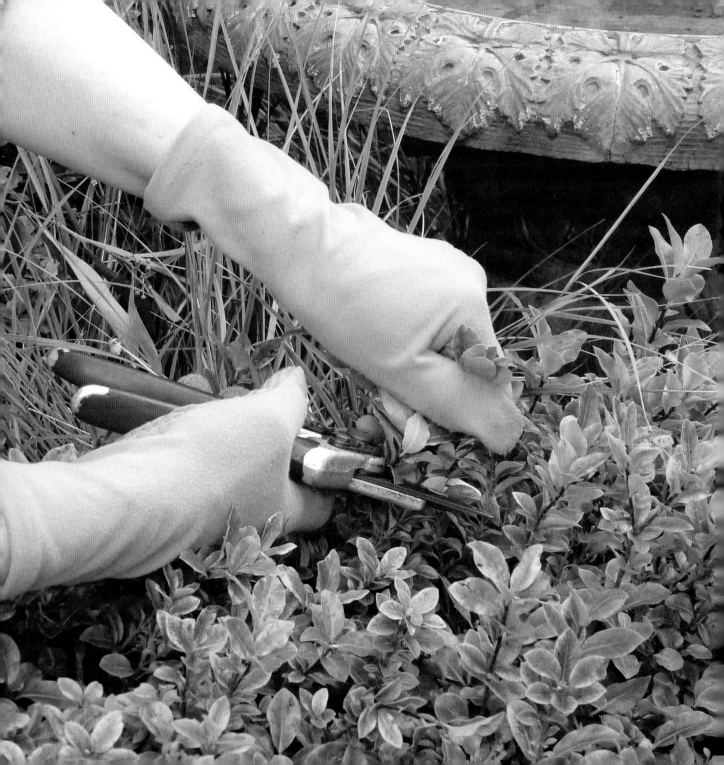

TWO

Balancing Act

*G*ood physical health calls for balance in many areas – muscle strength, nutrition, strong immune system, balance and coordination, hormone levels and good circulation. Cancer treatment can compromise many of these important functions, but fortunately, treatment has come a long way in recent years and we have ways of dealing with each challenge.

When my mother, Sue Nybro, was diagnosed with breast cancer in 1978, she became unable to continue her treatment due to a very low white blood count. Her doctors discontinued chemotherapy, and 10 years later, her cancer returned with a vengeance, ultimately taking her life. Now, she may have had a recurrence anyway – we can't know that – but what we know today just may have been enough to save her. The side effects that she experienced kept her from going outside and tending to her rose bushes, an activity we now know could have at least helped her quality of life.

Gardening isn't going to change the fact that you have cancer and that you need treatment, but with all the other challenges that can hitch a ride during treatment, your garden is ready to help alleviate some of your pain and discomfort – just be aware that the name of the game is doing it *safely*.

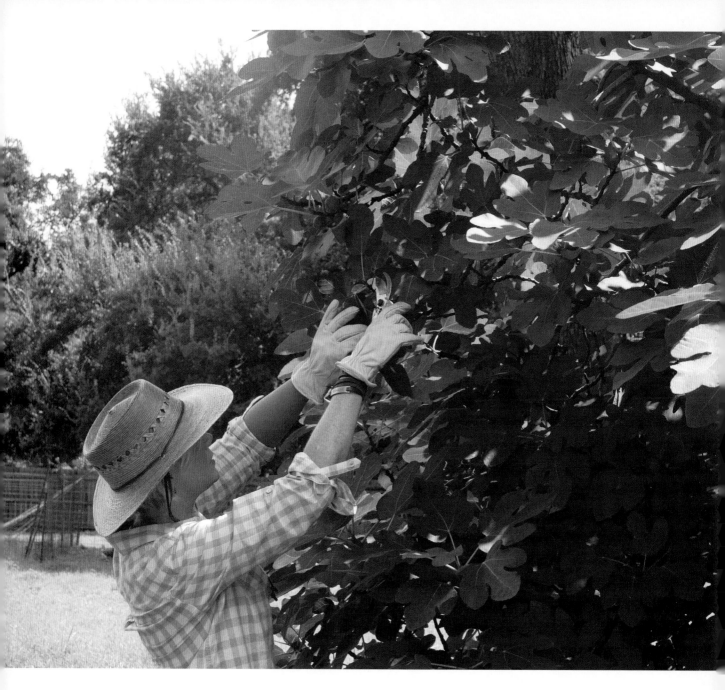

Nerve Damage

As I was finishing up chemotherapy, I began to have a tingly, numbing sensation in my fingertips, toes and balls of my feet. My oncologist told me that this could happen – it's called peripheral neuropathy, and it can cause a lot more problems than simply the odd sensations. When your nerves are damaged or even destroyed from surgery or treatment, your risks of falling, burning and cutting yourself ratchet up.

As gardeners, we know that all different parts of our bodies are called into action

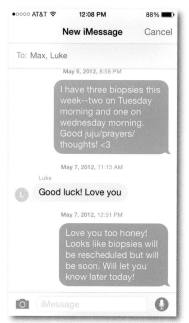

when we go outside to garden. And I'll bet that most of us have injured ourselves in the process – and that's probably even *before* we went through treatment. So take the proper precautions to protect yourself. Like it or not, your body is different right now, and safety, although always important, is now paramount.

If you have nerve damage in your fingers, you can easily accidentally cut yourself with pruners, shears or saws, so be sure to wear sturdy gloves. I like

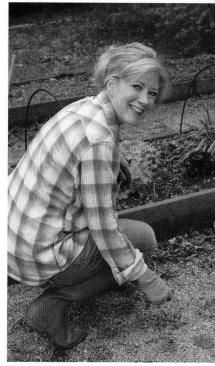

I was a stickler about proper garden gear even before my diagnosis!

gloves that have the rubberized palms for gripping tools and keeping my hands dry, but leather gloves will work well, too. Also, watch out for water that has been sitting in a hose and has heated up in the sun – you can burn yourself without even realizing it.

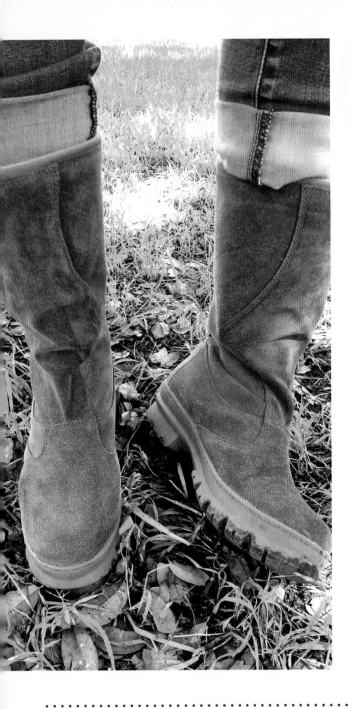

Safety Tips for Nerve Damage/Balance Issues

- Wear sturdy closed-toe shoes, preferably with lug soles, no flip-flops or sandals.
- Always wear protective gloves.
- Buy ergonomic tools for easier grip (see Resources section at back of book).
- Leave more potentially dangerous activities (sawing, electric hand tools) to someone else, at least for the time being.
- Garden during full daylight hours.
- Bring flashlight and/or companion if you need to go out to the garden after dark.
- Construct raised beds with seating ledges from 8-18" W x 18-24" H.
- Make sure garden paths are smooth, level and firm, and with good traction.
- Pathways should be 3-4' wide.
- Pathway/ground grade should not exceed 8% (this means no super-sloping paths).
- If your property is sloped, create a tiered pathway system for stability.

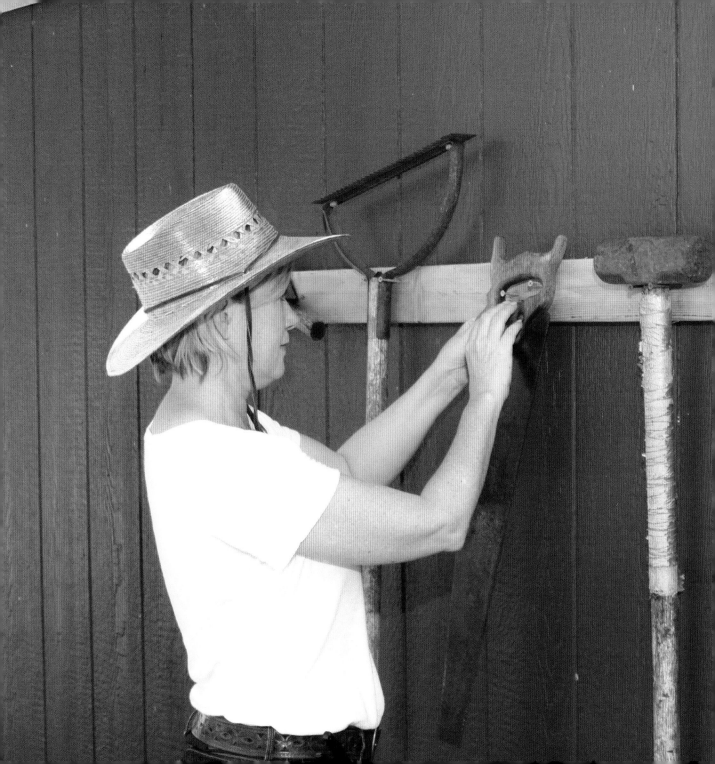

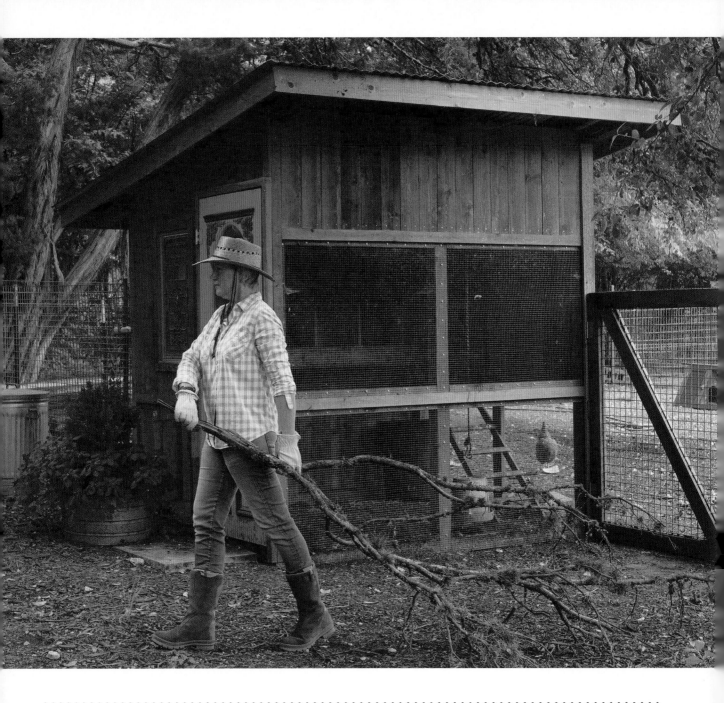

I was fortunate that the neuropathy in my fingers cleared up pretty quickly after ending chemotherapy – that's good news for a writer – but the nerve damage in my feet has lingered right up to the present, and that's kind of bad news for a gardener. However, I've learned how to compensate. To be fair, it's improved quite a bit. I don't fall anymore, tripping is at a minimum, and I really only notice it at night when I'm walking on uneven ground. So, I don't do that, and if I have to, I bring someone along with me.

Circulation

Most people don't feel too well as they are going through treatment – while some make it through with few side affects or lingering issues, others experience a wider range of struggles. When you're not feeling well, you tend to be more sedentary – lying on the couch and watching TV, sitting in the recliner with your feet up, or curling up in bed for the day. Look, sometimes those things are going to happen, and sometimes they need to happen. But understand that an overall sedentary lifestyle with a lack of movement can lead to many new problems and exacerbate existing ones.

Circulation issues, heart problems, blood clots, breathing problems, increased weight, high blood pressure, mood disturbances and increased risk of certain cancers are all related to sedentary lifestyles. I understand that we are talking about being sedentary during treatment as opposed to having a lifelong habit of this, but it's still not good for you. And if you have problems with lymphedema as a result of your surgery or treatment, lack of movement can make that problem much, much worse (I found that one out the hard way).

My lymphedema, for months after my diagnosis of it, was not responding too well to rehab. I even attended rehab twice a week for the first few months, and that

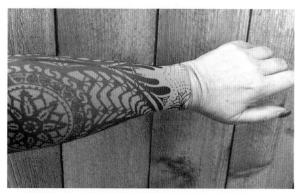

I wear compression sleeves to protect my arm while working out or gardening. Fun sleeves like this one are from the LympheDiva company (see Resources).

stubborn swelling just wouldn't go down. I do credit my wonderful rehab therapists, Jackie, Rhonda and Ellen, for maintaining the swelling so that it didn't *increase*, but we were all frustrated because we weren't hitting our goals for my arm very quickly.

When I got the green light to start with some light yoga, it was amazing how my arm responded. Now, yoga might not be your thing, but the point is to find something to do that gets your circulation flowing through your body – your overall healing depends upon it.

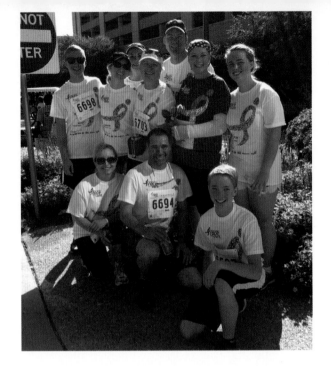

Good circulation helps with:

● Distributing blood, oxygen, nutrients and lymph fluids throughout the body
● Focusing the brain
● Bringing color to your skin
● Removing toxins and lactic acid
● Promoting muscle tone
● Keeping us healthy and feeling lively
● Tissue healing

So let's get up and get moving. I am not encouraging you to run a marathon right now; I'm not even talking about race-walking. I'm just talking about moving, where your feet are on the ground and your head is above your feet. Go outside into your garden, walk around, shuffle if you need to, and swing your arms. Getting your heart rate up a bit is a plus, but if you promise me to simply get outside and move once a day, I'll take that. If you are further along in your recovery, walk around the block or better yet, join a team and walk a cancer-funding 10k.

My family and I did the Komen Race for the Cure right after I finished chemotherapy and before I started radiation. I looked like a wounded warrior – bald head, my left arm bandaged for lymphedema treatment, balance all wonky –

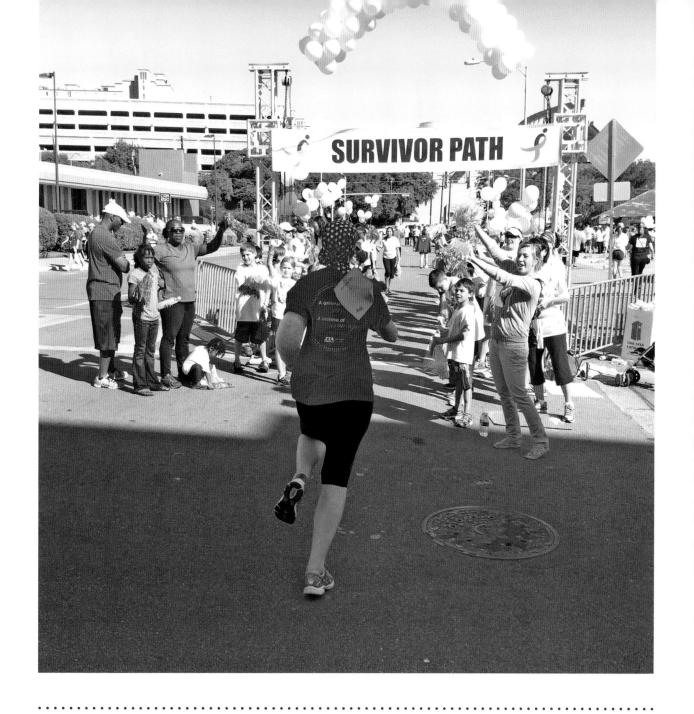

and in fact, my niece Christine burst into tears when she saw me. But we all got through it, had a great time walking the race, and I felt wonderful and invigorated afterwards.

Your oncologist or surgeon will have given you post-treatment and post-op instructions, and you should adhere to them to a T. And I'm betting that neither of them wrote, "Sit on your butt for an entire month and eat Doritos. Better yet, order pizza and have it delivered to your recliner. You deserve it." You can't fool me; I know they did not tell you this. There is a reason that, even if you are kept in the hospital for several days after your surgery, the nursing staff gets you out of that bed and walking around the floor as soon as humanly possible.

Another possible issue can happen with some post-treatment medications. I take one that can increase my risk of developing blood clots, so it's very important for me to keep moving and active.

Still worried you don't have the energy? You'll have more after you get up and move, but here's a way to do it gently if you are just starting out and need to take baby steps (literally):

If you've been sitting or lying down for long, gently wiggle your toes and start to move your feet and hands. Don't jump up quickly from a position or pose you've held for a long time, as you could pull a muscle or lose your balance.

- Take a few deep breaths.
- Stretch your limbs and pull your arms over your head (assuming your range of motion will allow that or you do not have stitches to worry about).
- Slowly get up from your seated/lying-down position, and have assistance if necessary.
- Gently and carefully go outside and walk around, even for 5 or 10 minutes.

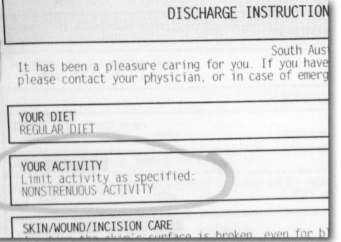

DISCHARGE INSTRUCTION

South Aus

It has been a pleasure caring for you. If you have please contact your physician, or in case of emerg

YOUR DIET
REGULAR DIET

YOUR ACTIVITY
Limit activity as specified:
NONSTRENUOUS ACTIVITY

SKIN/WOUND/INCISION CARE

It says 'nonstrenuous activity', not 'no' activity!

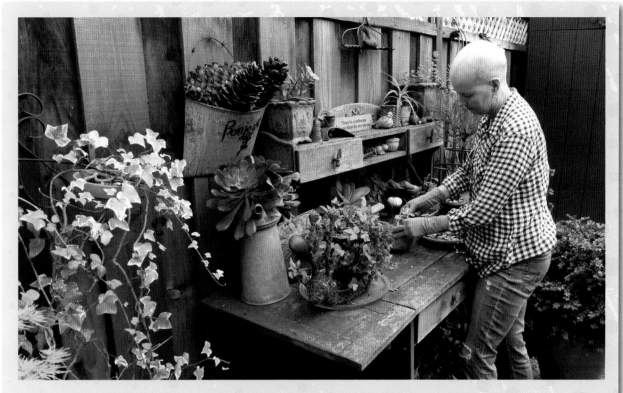

Garden Activities for Circulation

- Yoga, particularly with inverted poses or asanas
- Reaching overhead to prune or harvest
- Swinging arms while walking through garden
- Light stretching on your patio, deck or in your garden
- Alternating poses in garden – standing, bending, reaching, squatting – using rails, a companion/helper or cane/walker to steady yourself if necessary
- Potting small plants (a number of different actions required)

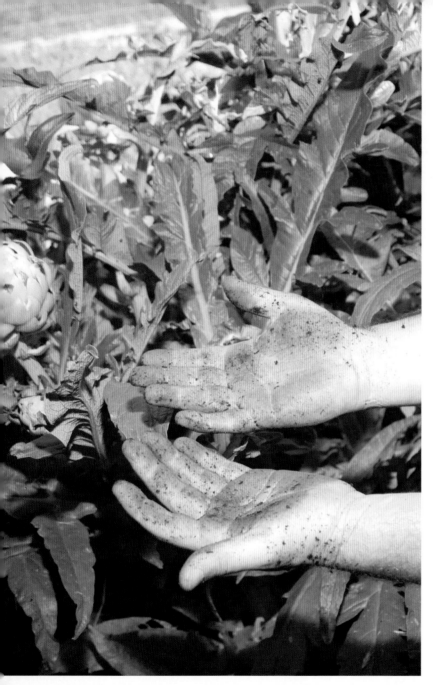

Immune System, Hormones & Body Chemistry

Bacteria have gotten a bum rap in recent years. We've become so "clean" conscious with all of our antibacterial cleaners, disinfectants, using bleach on all surfaces, and washing hands that we forget that not all bacteria are created equal. Now, don't get me wrong – I am not advocating throwing caution to the wind, particularly for those of you who are immunosuppressed. That would not only be foolish, it could be dangerous.

Nature, however, exposes us to what scientists call "old friend" organisms that are not only good for us, they increase our bodies' probiotics and give our immune systems a jolt. Specifically, we're talking about *Mycobacterium vaccae*, a harmless bacteria commonly found in soil. *M. vaccae* increases the release and metabolism of serotonin in the parts of the brain

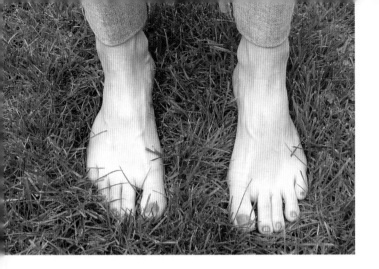

that control mood and cognitive function. While *M. vaccae* may not have the same direct effect as taking an antidepressant medication, gardening is a natural way to introduce this good bacteria into our systems.

Many studies have shown that simply walking through your garden and inhaling can trigger exposure, so actually working in the soil (digging, weeding, hoeing, shoveling) can work wonders. Similarly, light and short periods of sun exposure can increase Vitamin D levels, leading to increased serotonin (important for calmness and emotional well-being) and dopamine (important for attention, motivation and goal-directed behavior). It's important to note, however, that you can still cover

up to protect your skin and hands while enjoying the benefits of these activities – it's not necessary to sacrifice one to gain the other.

After checking with your oncologist, it's probably safe to dig around in the soil without gloves on occasion – or even walk barefoot sometimes – to expose yourself to "good bacteria," but if you have any cuts or open sores, it's best to be cautious and put the gloves and shoes back on!

While I was going through treatment, my oncologist encouraged me to work outside in the garden. First, he knew it was what I did for a living, but more importantly, he knew it was what I did for pleasure. There was only one week during treatment when I became severely neutropenic (extremely low white blood count) and could not work in the garden at all because I was hospitalized and my immune system

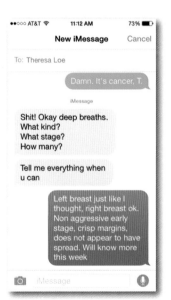

Soil Safety Tip

When digging in the soil or bringing in compost, make sure it is clean, high quality material (preferably organic). Avoid any soil or compost that was made with waste (from composting toilets, for example). In our area we have a material called "Dillo Dirt" that is wonderful for many applications, but it's made at waste water treatment plants, which can introduce potentially unsafe bacteria for those who are immunosuppressed.

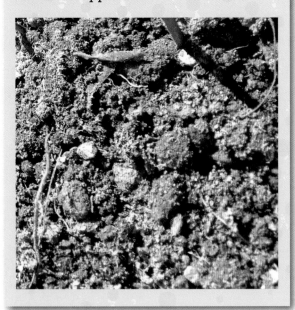

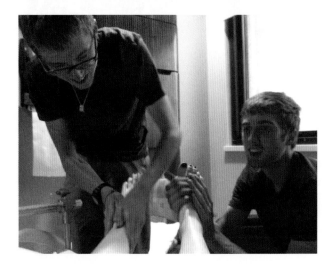

was so compromised, but after that, I was given instructions to double-glove (use sterile surgical gloves underneath my garden gloves) and have at it! And before you start to feel sorry for me that I was popped back in the hospital, take a look at these hooligans I call my sons – I was treated with a visit from Max and Luke and got a foot rub out of it.

The lesson here is to have safety in mind first. If you have been used to being a Weekend Warrior, a devil-may-care gardener or have a "Bring it on!" kind of personality, consider what your body has been through and adjust your activities accordingly. To do anything less could create more problems than it's possibly worth. ∾

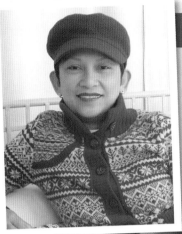

Survivor Spotlight

Name: Mimi

Age at diagnosis: 38

Diagnosis: Breast Cancer (Invasive Ductal Carcinoma)

Stage: 1

Tip: Dance morning, noon and night – even in the garden as you're weeding or watering! – it does your body good and your spirit even better!

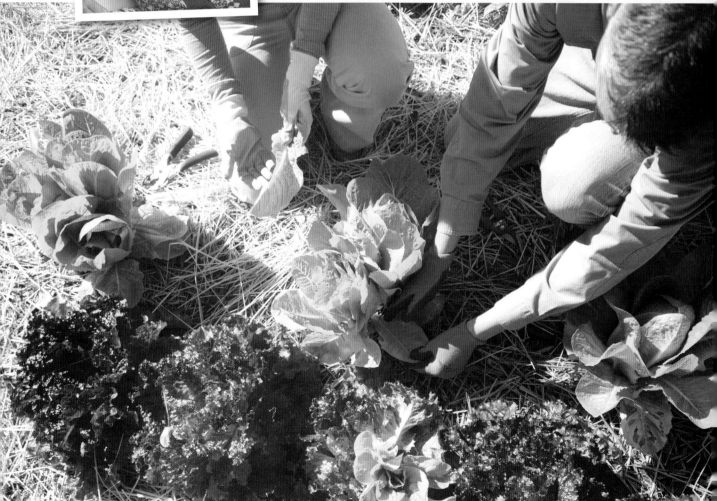

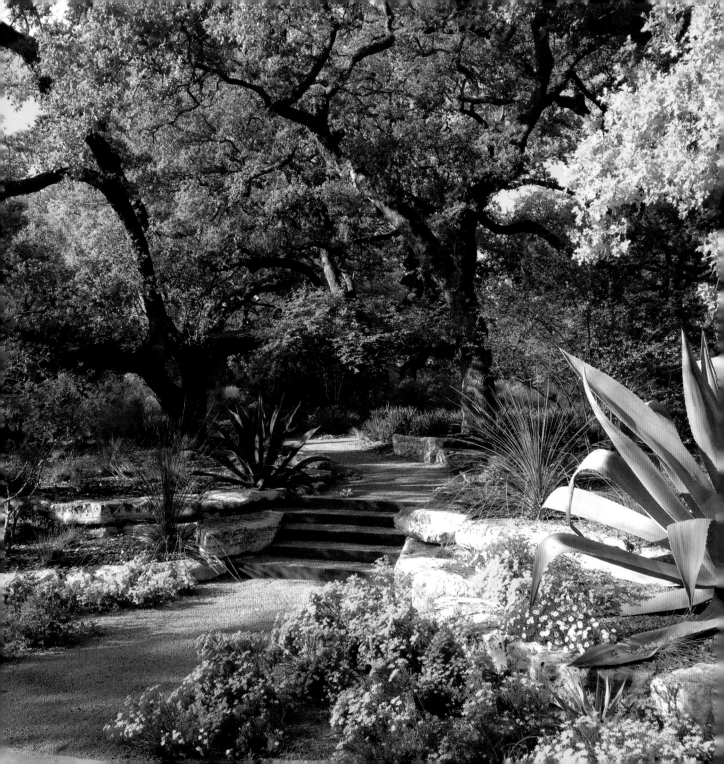

THREE

Therapeutic Gardens

While writing this book, I made a quick trip out to MD Anderson Cancer Center in Houston, Texas. It's only about a 3-hour drive, and I'd heard so many good things about their gardens from friends who had sought treatment there, so I wanted to see it for myself. I was fortunate to be given a personal tour by the facilities manager, David Renninger, who is responsible for many of the center's landscape decisions in recent years.

I'm not really sure what I was expecting – I know how my own garden has helped in my personal healing, but I wasn't sure how a large institution like MD Anderson would interpret what is healing for those going through cancer treatment. David showed me a prairie planting that featured dozens of native plants, a vegetable and herb garden, a room where cooking classes are given, formal knot gardens, a paved labyrinth, a butterfly garden and beautifully appointed sitting gardens on various terraces. There was attention to color, scent, placement and texture – and the gardens as a whole were delightfully different from most institutional landscapes.

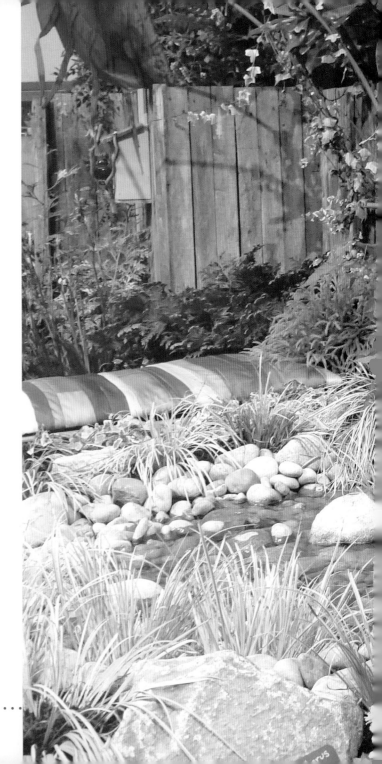

Although it's going through some changes with current construction at the hospital, MD Anderson also has an extensive rose garden that allows roses to be cut and brought into some patients' rooms. For those who can't get outside to enjoy the fresh air and walk the lovely and peaceful paths through the outside gardens, that little bit of nature delivered in a scented form can be such an important part of connecting with the outside world.

As I walked these beautiful gardens, I began to wonder about what makes a "therapeutic" garden different from a regular old pretty garden, so when I returned home I asked my friend Naomi Sachs to weigh in. Naomi and I have been friends and colleagues for several years. She is the founding director of the Therapeutic Landscapes Network, a knowledge base and gathering space that provides information, education, advocacy and inspiration about landscapes that promote health and well-being – and she recently co-authored the book *Therapeutic Landscapes: An Evidence-Based Approach to Designing Healing Gardens and Restorative Outdoor Spaces.* I know – I pick impressive people to hang with, don't I?

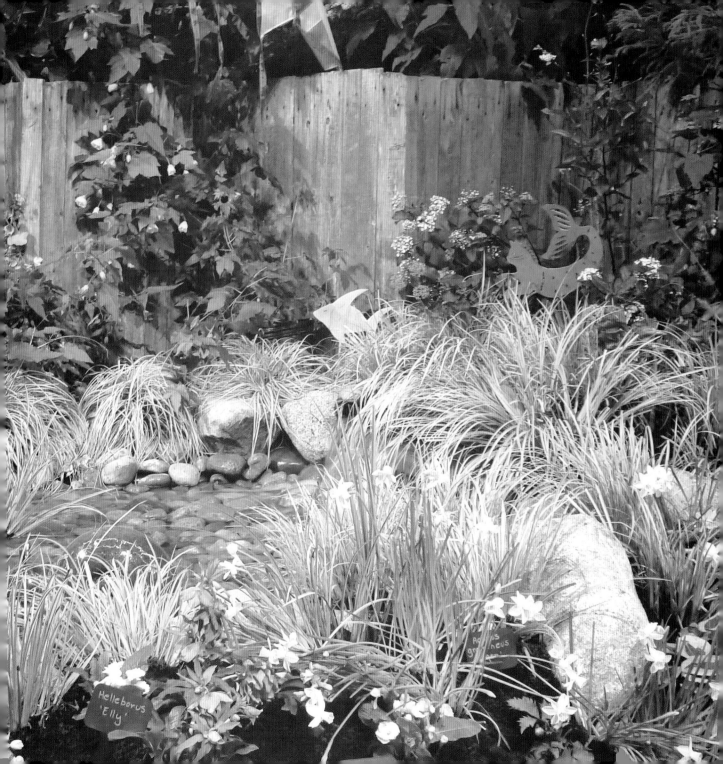

Helleborus
'Elly'

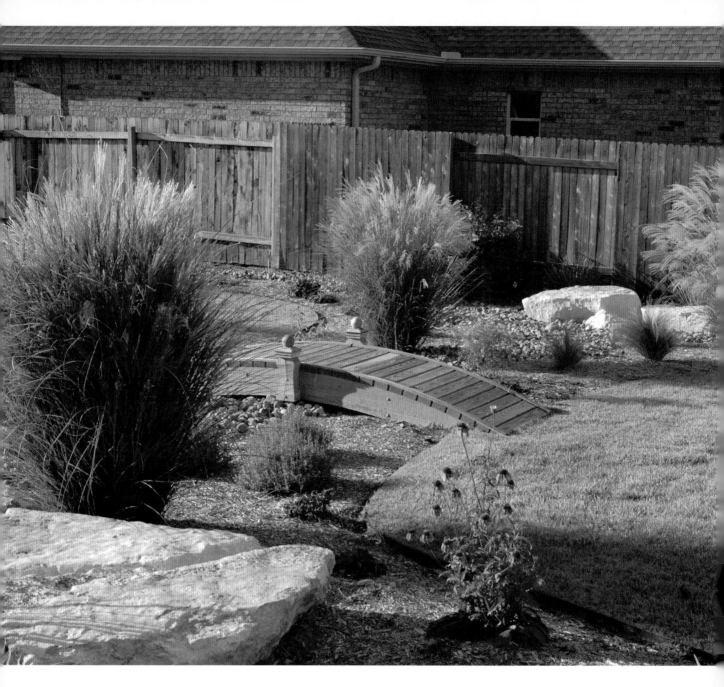

"Many times institutional healing gardens are as much for the family and friends as they are for the people receiving treatment," Naomi says. "There is attention to providing shade, opportunities for walking, areas to relax – or there may even be a 'viewing garden' next to infusion rooms so people can enjoy a beautiful scene." She says scent can be a great thing for some patients, but not all, as many people going through treatment are sensitive to smells and odors.

"The garden must be carefully planned and maintained to reduce the risk of infection from bacteria in plants, water, and animal droppings," she says, "as people in treatment often have compromised immune systems and need to avoid the risk of infection."

I asked Naomi to name two easy things a home gardener can do to make their own space more therapeutic.

"One, give yourself what brings you joy; and two, don't try to do too much! At home, I think the most important question is, 'What will make my heart sing?' Of course, this is an important question for any home gardener, but it's especially critical for someone who is dealing with a lot of physical and emotional stress.

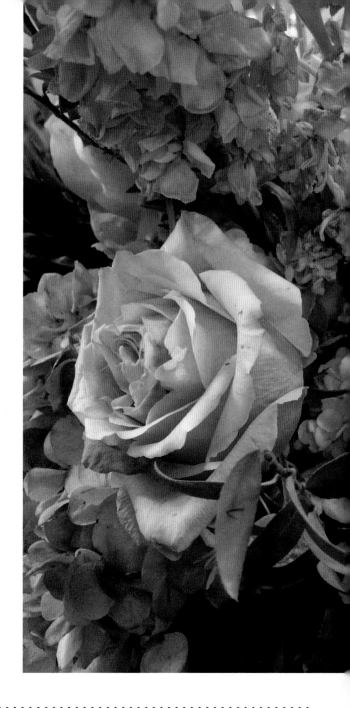

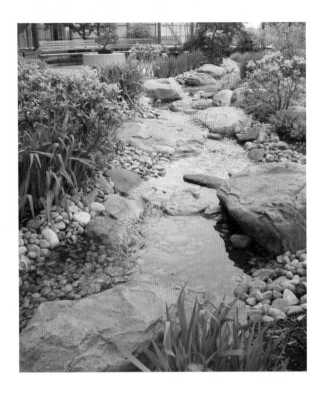

Really think about what will bring you joy. Is it seeing a riot of color? Maybe plant a lot of annuals that will give that big boost. Don't worry about planning the perfect perennial border! Save that for when you're feeling better. Or maybe you do want to think about the long term: Plant a tree, something you know will last more than a hundred years. If the weeds are getting you down and you just. don't. have. the energy...then ask someone for help, or hire someone to pull those weeds.

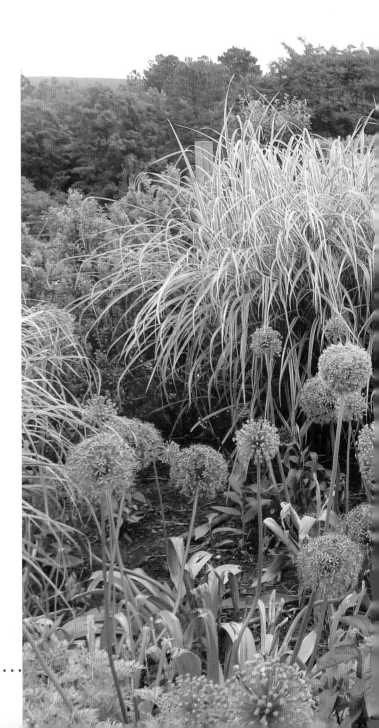

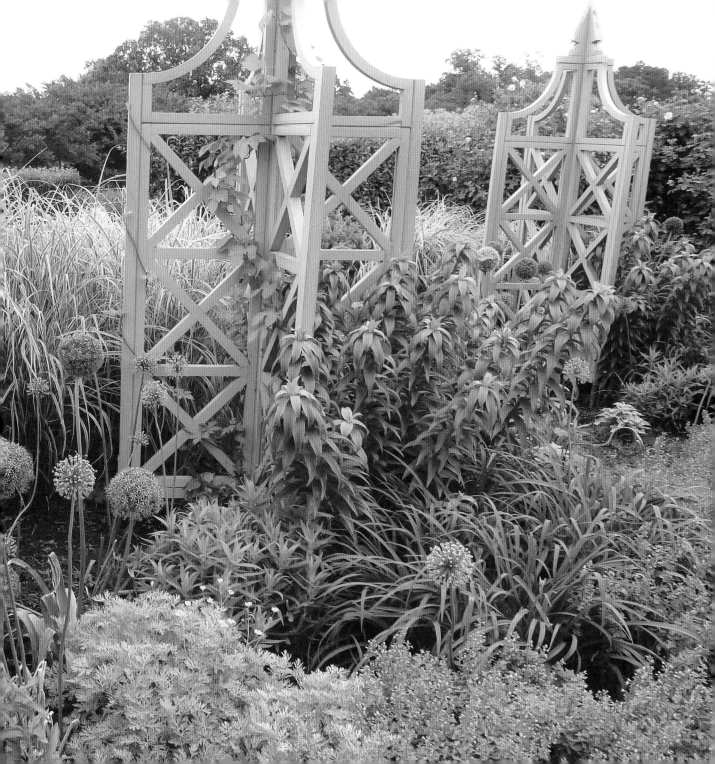

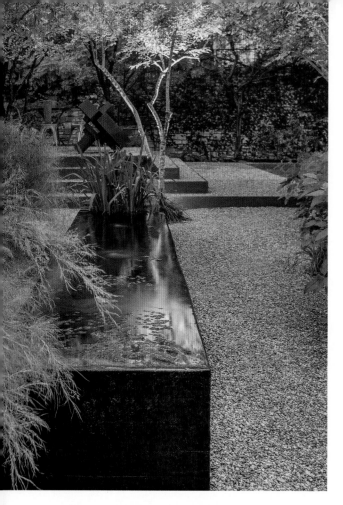

underneath, and you've got an instant 24/7 garden room. In other words, listen to your heart and follow it!"

● ● ●

I've also recently become acquainted with renowned landscape architect Christy Ten Eyck, who designs public and private spaces of healing. Her projects have included hospitals, schools, city streets and private residences – and she says that healing spaces, regardless of where they are, have something in common. "When you engage two or more of the senses simultaneously," she explains, "your heart rate slows, your blood pressure drops and you begin to feel more relaxed and calm."

So, even though places like MD Anderson are, for obvious reasons, inter-ested in healing gardens on an institu-tional level, Naomi and Christy show us that we can attain the same sense of relaxation, healing and calm in our own personal gardens. Surround yourself with what you love, don't try to do too much, and appeal to two or more senses – and remember Naomi's wise words: "Listen to your heart and follow it!" ~

"Maybe just being outside – by your-self, or with family and friends – is the most important thing, but you've only got a deck, or a lawn with no shade. Then perhaps the best 'therapeutic garden element' you can have is one of those cloth shade canopies. String some lights

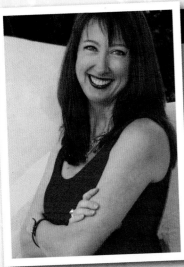

Survivor Spotlight

Name: Lisa

Diagnosis: DCIS (Ductal Carcinoma In-Situ) and IDC (Invasive Ductal Carcinoma)

Age at diagnosis: 41 and 43

Stage: 1

Tip: I find it more healing than most anything else to be in nature and watch the river flow. At night, the fireflies take over and they bring an indescribable calming effect (or maybe that is the wine). Sometimes you don't have to actually garden at all; just being outside and a part of nature is exactly what you need.

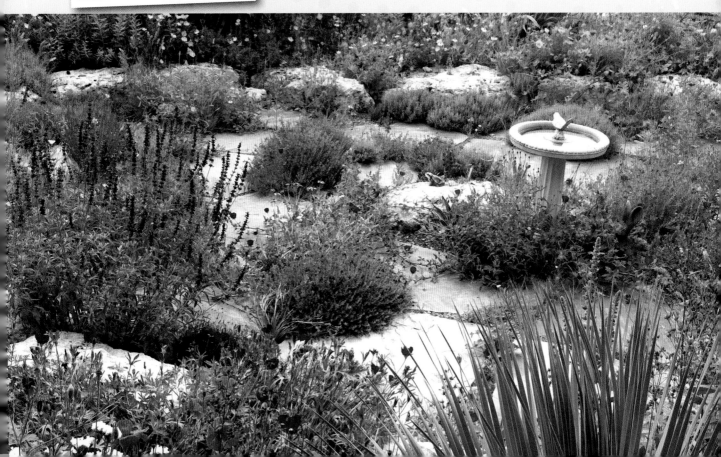

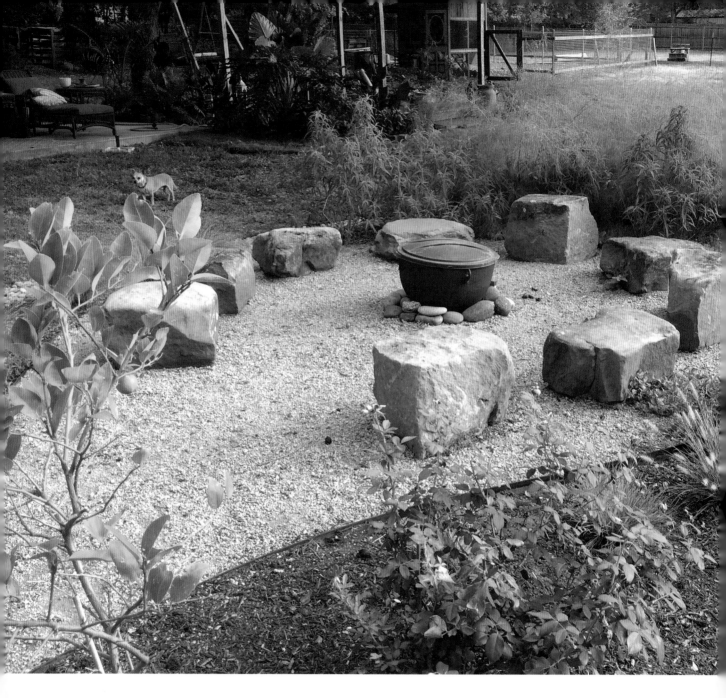

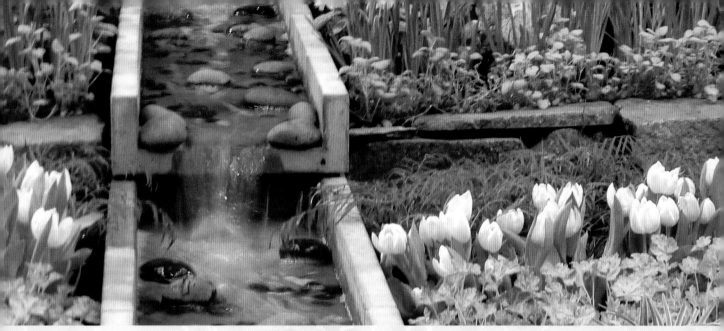

Survivor Spotlight

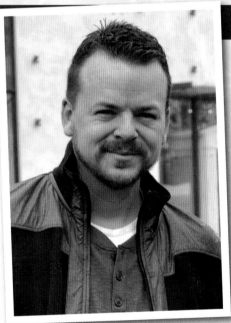

Name: Nathan

Age at diagnosis: 36

Diagnosis: Head and Neck Cancer
(Squamous-cell Carcinoma)

Stage: 4

Tip: Live, don't just exist. Lose yourself in nature to discover your inner peace. Becoming one with the natural world helps to heal the body and mind and offers a sense of meaning and purpose. For me, it's the solitude of being away exploring the vast deserts of the Southwest. I cannot imagine a more profound way to allow my body and soul to heal as I continue down my path of life. So find your inner peace. Relax, breathe, laugh and live. Live the life you were created for and each day as if it were your last.

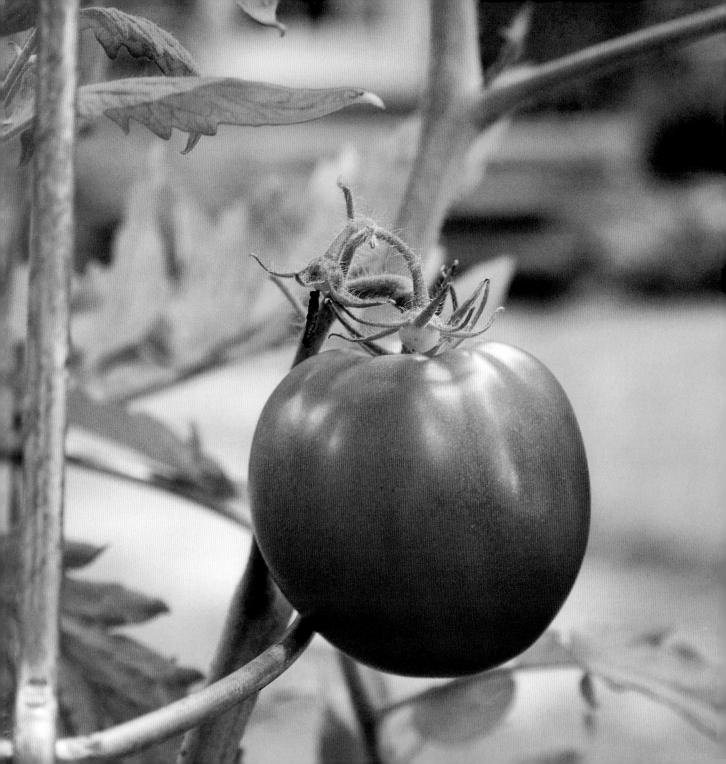

FOUR

Food is Good Medicine...
to strengthen, heal, calm and invigorate

*G*ood nutrition is, of course, always important, but even more so as you are going through cancer treatment and recovering afterwards. And recovery can take several years, so the kinder you are to your body, the better. Now, I'm betting you've had some of the same experiences I have – after my cancer diagnosis, I had a stream of emails, text messages and Facebook messages with all sorts of well-meaning advice on diets and food that would heal or cure. Frozen cottage cheese, no sugar, odd combinations of foods, foods I couldn't even pronounce – and while I

was thankful everybody was thinking of me, there was no way I could figure out which one of these things was best, and I felt so overwhelmed I wanted to scream. (Instead, I began making my fiancé field all of those messages for me. The man deserves some sort of medal or angel wings.) I won't be making any drastic dietary recommendations to you; my best advice is to work with your doctor or a dietician who is experienced in dealing with people in cancer treatment, and then to use a good dose of common sense.

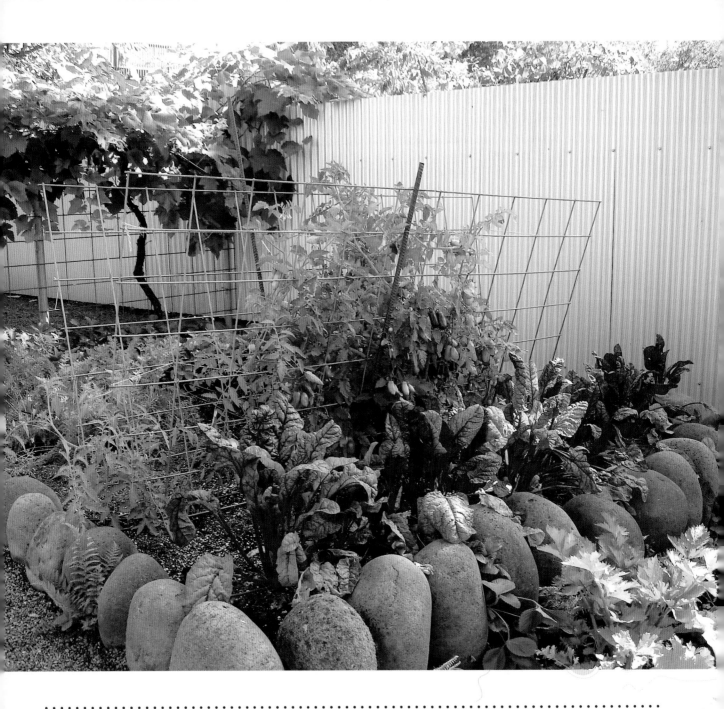

That being said, your garden can be your best source of healthy food for you as you recover and regain your strength, so stock up on those seed packets and small transplants and get out in the garden!

What Food is the Healthiest?

Cancer treatment can cause many problems that affect your ability to eat, stay nourished and feel strong – mouth sores, upset stomach, changes in taste/smell, vomiting, diarrhea/constipation, sore throat and loss of appetite make it very difficult for you to stay healthy and strong when you need it the most. If you're experiencing many of these problems, your doctor will probably advise you to simply eat what you are able to keep down, but beyond that, there are a number of common sense guidelines to healthy eating during this time:

- Choose organic foods as much as possible.
- Limit processed foods like fast food or foods that come in cans or bags.
- Stay hydrated with water and decaffeinated tea.

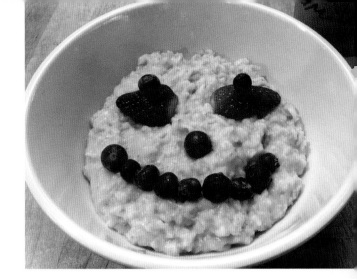

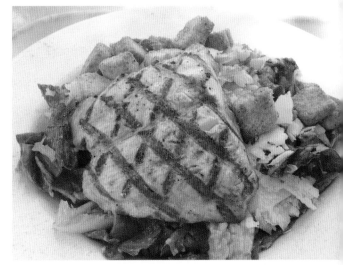

- Maintain good protein intake for strength.
- Increase your vegetables and fruits, particularly leafy greens.

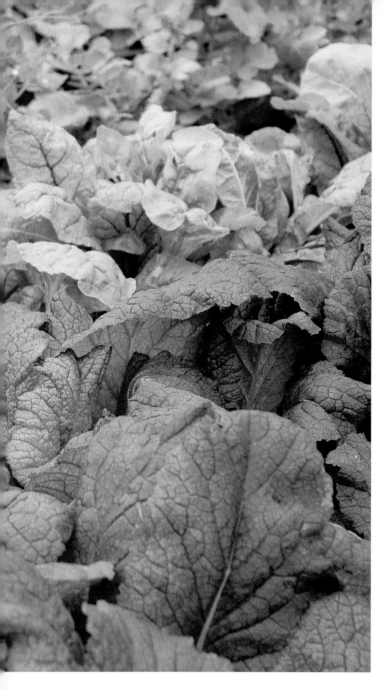

The last bullet point is, of course, where your garden can be of tremendous help to you. Growing organic fruits, herbs and vegetables in your own garden is much less expensive than buying them at the store, and nearly anyone anywhere can grow them. And no worries if you don't already have a vegetable garden – simply tuck your broccoli, kale and tomato plants in with your flowers and shrubs, assuming they are all getting the appropriate amounts of sunlight and water. Combined gardens like these are not only beautiful but practical as well. Before I was diagnosed, I lived in an apartment where I balcony gardened, and I often planted lettuces right next to the flowers in my hayrack planters. I have a full acre on which to garden now.

Look for easy-to-grow foods that are simple to prepare and soothing to eat, avoiding anything spicy like jalepeno peppers, particularly if you have mouth sores. Green and red bell peppers are wonderful when combined with other produce in juices, toning down the potential for mouth irritation.

Veggies, Fruits & Herbs for Treatment Strength

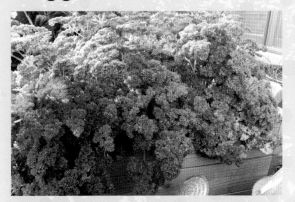
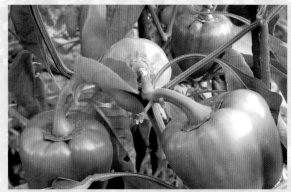
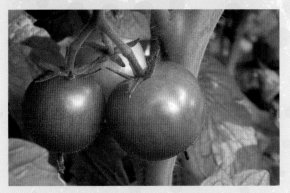
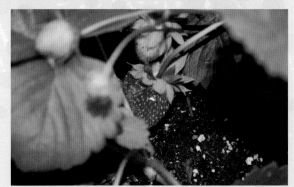

- Greens: kale, spinach, collards, lettuce, Swiss chard, beets (both the root and the greens)
- Tomatoes
- Bell peppers
- All squashes: yellow, zucchini, acorn, spaghetti

- All herbs: mint, parsley, basil, rosemary, chamomile, lavender, thyme
- Citrus: lemon, lime, grapefruit, orange
- Berries: strawberries, blueberries, blackberries, raspberries

Green Drinks & Smoothies

Most doctors and nutritionists agree that healthy smoothies and green drinks are good for you, but please be careful – during cancer treatment is generally not the best time to go on a juice cleanse or diet. Rather, use smoothies and green drinks as a snack or as a healthy way to keep calories and nutrients down when your system is in revolt. These drinks are also very soothing for sore mouths and upset stomachs, with their creamy textures and cool temperatures.

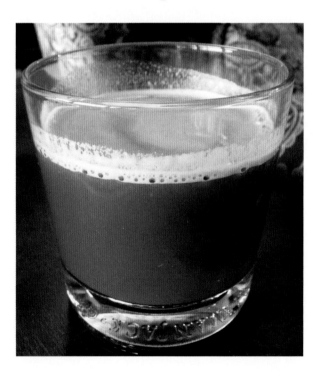

I like to alternate with smoothies and juices, as smoothies retain all the valuable fiber in your ingredients, but juices take an enormous amount of ingredients and their nutrients and turn them into an extracted juice. It would be difficult to eat the amount of greens, vegetables and fruits that go into making one serving of juice.

Basic Smoothie Recipe Using a Blender

Good quality blenders take your ingredients and blend them together very finely. You don't necessarily need a $500 blender, but the really inexpensive ones may struggle to adequately blend your ingredients, and the motor may actually burn up. Mine cost about $100 and I've been using it for about 3 years to make very creamy smoothies.

Start with your liquid, then add a banana and any other fruits and leafy greens you want (frozen fruits add a frosty coolness to the drink), and finish with any add-ins to increase your protein intake. Go easy on the acidic fruits like pineapple if you are experiencing mouth sores, opting for soothing berries instead.

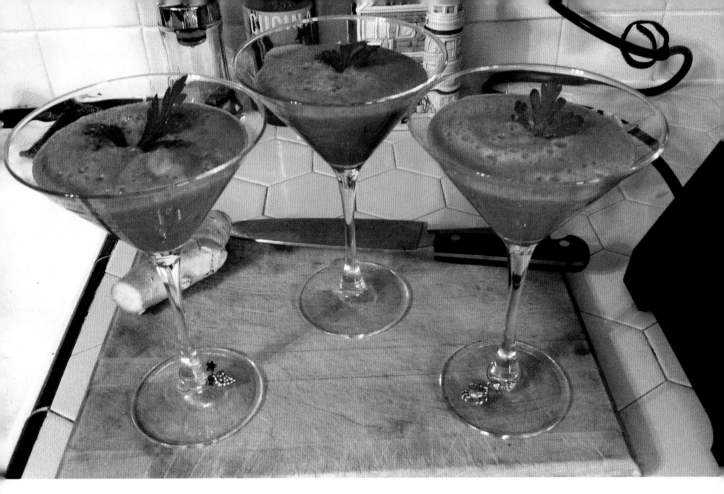

Liquids	Fruits	Greens	Add-Ins
Almond milk	Strawberries	Kale	Chia seeds
Coconut milk	Bananas	Spinach	Protein powder
Soy milk	Blueberries	Romaine	Hemp seeds
Fruit juice	Blackberries	Swiss chard	Greek yogurt
Coconut water	Mangoes	Collard	Oatmeal
Water	Pineapple	Beet	Nut butters

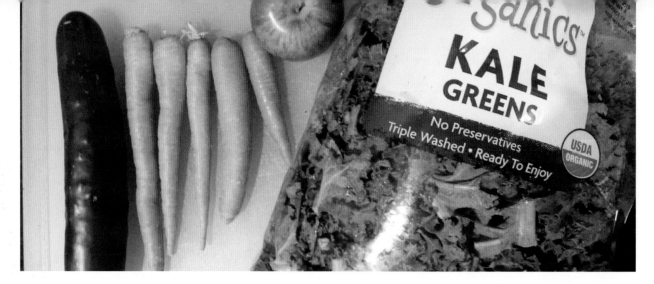

Green Drink Combos Using a Juicer

No juicer is truly inexpensive, because the machine is actually extracting the liquid from the produce. This is more of an investment, but well worth it if your budget allows. I didn't purchase one myself – I use our housemate's juicer, but I typically make enough for everyone in the household. If you have some of the ingredients in your garden (spinach, beets and kale, for example), you'll be ahead of the game, but if you need to buy all the ingredients at the grocery store, it'll take about $20 to make enough juice for a couple of days. I personally can't afford to do this daily unless I grow most of the produce myself.

Run each ingredient through the juicer until you get your desired amount of liquid. I like to alternate ingredients so that I know I'm getting a balance of tastes as the juices are extracted. The leftover pulp or fiber can be composted or fed to your chickens if you have them (mine devour it).

Good Juicing Combos

Kale, apple, carrot
Spinach, pear, apple
Kale, cucumber, grapes, apple
Ginger, beet, carrot, apple
Beet, carrots, spinach
Kale, spinach, cucumber, ginger
Spinach, cucumber, apple
Spinach, bell peppers, apple

Aromatherapy to the Rescue

Fragrance has long been known to excite, calm, invigorate, soothe and relax – and the fragrances from plants in your garden can be the best and easiest ones to use. But which plants do what, and what are the best ways to use them? My goal is always to do what is the easiest yet most effective. I'll spend a good deal of time on something if I know that the reward will be great, but frankly, I didn't have the energy when I was going through chemotherapy. So let's keep it simple, shall we? Here's a list of common ailments related to cancer treatment, and fragrances known to soothe them.

Scents & Their Uses

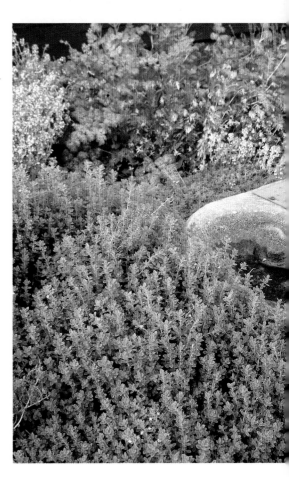

AILMENT	FRAGRANT PLANT
Anxiety	Basil, bergamot, cedarwood, hyssop, patchouli, ylang–ylang
Concentration	Basil, rosemary
Constipation	Fennel
Depression	Camphor, bergamot, jasmine, juniper, thyme, clary sage
Diarrhea	Eucalyptus, chamomile
Digestion	Cinnamon, lemongrass, rose, rosemary, basil, chamomile
Fatigue	Peppermint, rosemary, sage, lavender, thyme
Headaches	Basil, marjoram, lavender, peppermint, rose, rosemary, thyme
Insomnia	Camphor, lavender, clary sage
Mouth sores	Clove
Nausea	Fennel, sandlewood
Neuralgia	Clove, Melissa (lemon balm)
Skin sores	Clove, juniper
Stress	Rose, lavender

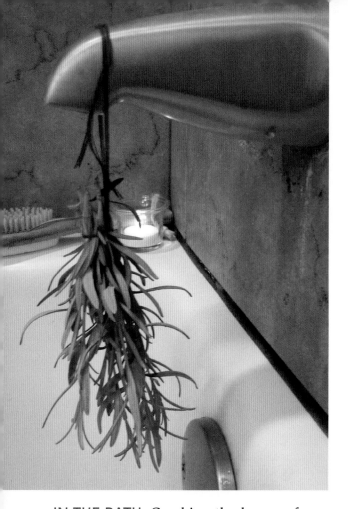

AT BEDTIME: Tuck the leaves of calming herbs into a small cloth bag and slip it into your pillowcase. Good choices would be lavender and chamomile.

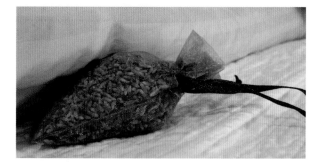

ON THE STOVETOP: Combine your plants in a small pot with water, bring to a boil and then turn the heat down to simmer. Add water as necessary. This is just like when you use oranges, cinnamon sticks and cloves on the stovetop to create a delicious-smelling potpourri at Christmastime.

IN THE BATH: Combine the leaves of your plants in a small cloth bag (use cheesecloth or muslin) – or simply tie into bundles – then float it in the water or hang it on the faucet to release the scents. Use the plants necessary to create the atmosphere you need – soothing, calming, relaxing or invigorating.

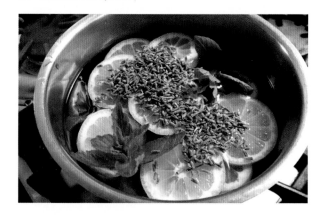

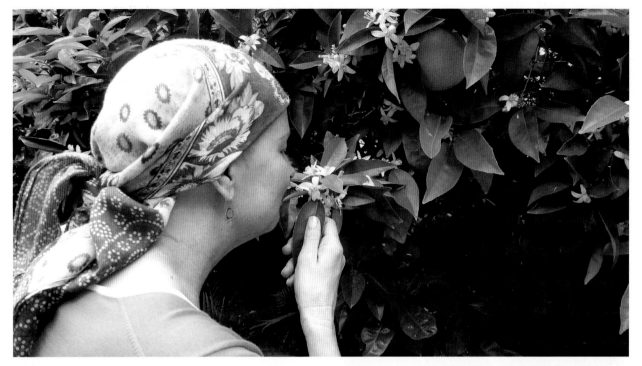

IN THE GARDEN: Simply walk through your garden and get up close to smell the leaves and petals. Pick some and crush them in your hand, then inhale deeply. I love doing this with rose petals, lemon thyme and mint.

BRING IT INSIDE: Those wonderfully scented flowers and herbs make beautiful arrangements indoors, on your dinner table or bedside. Go out into your garden and cut a few stems and sprigs, pop them in a vase or bud holder and enjoy their scent and beauty for days.

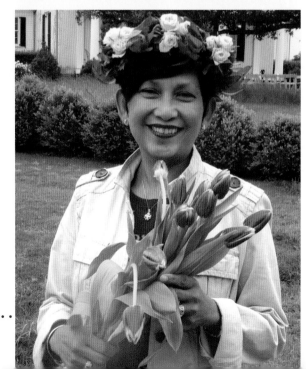

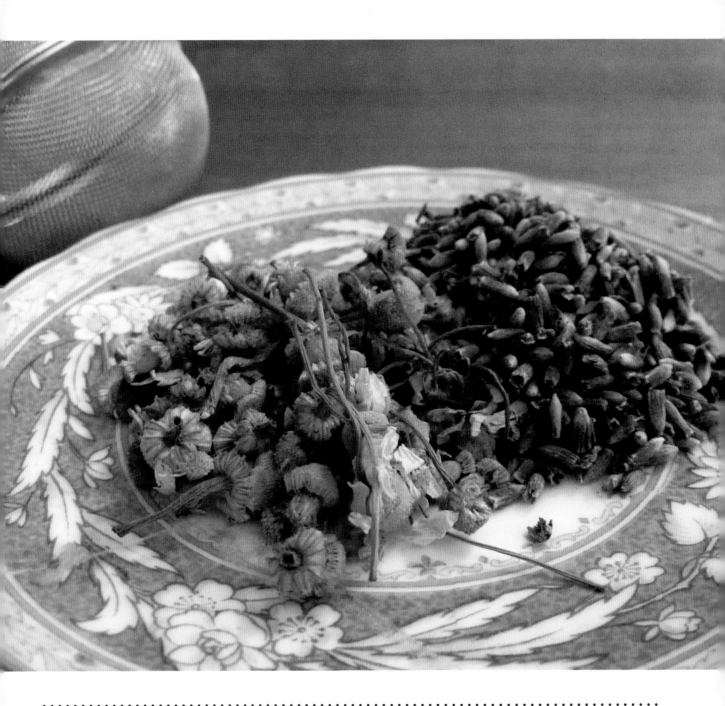

Soothing Herbal Remedies

As you're going through treatment, it's extremely important to check with your oncologist or primary care doctor before using any herbal supplement or treatment. I live in somewhat of a hippy town (Austin, Texas) where there are almost as many herb shops as there are Starbucks, but my oncologist warned me that even some natural herbs can work against your prescribed cancer medications – so please, please run everything you take past your doctor first. While my recommendations in this section use many of the same plants in the aromatherapy section, the difference is in the application. With aromatherapy, the gains are through the scent of the plant, but with herbal remedies and tinctures, the product is either ingested or applied to the skin.

GREEN TEA COMPRESS: When I was going through radiation, my radiation oncologist recommended that I steep some green tea, let it cool, then soak a washcloth in it to soothe my radiation burns. While you can certainly use store-bought green tea bags like I did, you can also use the leaves of *Camellia sinensis*. To be processed into a proper drinking tea, I'm sure the steps are much more complicated, but for a compress like the one here, steeping is just fine.

STEEPING TEA: Use 2 tablespoons of dried leaves or flowers or 4 tablespoons of fresh leaves or flowers to every 8 ounces of water for one serving of tea. Using the herb chart, combine plants to make your own recipe according to your need for calm, sleep, energy or headache relief. I like to use a tea ball with my leaves inside, or you can get an individual teapot with the infuser on the top.

HERBAL TINCTURES: Tinctures are concentrated liquid forms of herbs that are both easy to make and use. Gather together a glass jar with a lid, all of your chosen herbs, and alcohol, like vodka or rum (at least 80 proof). If you prefer to not use alcohol, you can substitute food grade vegetable glycerin or apple cider vinegar.

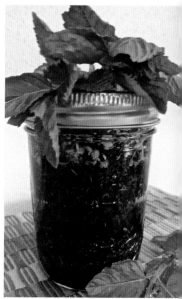

Mint and echinacea tincture for nausea

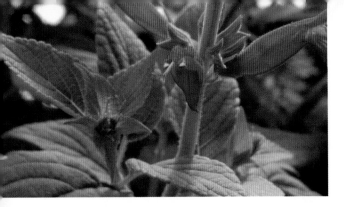

1/2 to 1 teaspoon up to three times a day. *Note:* Tinctures using apple cider need to be refrigerated, and tinctures made with glycerin have a slightly different finishing process (easily located through a quick Internet search).

Fill the jar 1/3 to 1/2 full with the herbs, add just enough boiling water to dampen the herbs and release their properties, and then fill the rest of the jar with alcohol, apple cider vinegar or vegetable glycerin. Give it a good stir, put the lid on, and keep in a cool and dry place, shaking daily, for about 6 weeks. Strain the herbs out, then use the tincture at a dose of

Herb Safety

- Obtain doctor's approval
- Research herbs for tinctures
- Obtain doctor's approval
- Research dosage & application
- Never harvest unknown plants
- Seriously... obtain doctor's approval

Survivor Spotlight

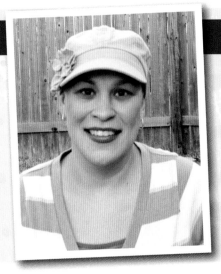

Name: Marisol

Age at diagnosis: 38

Diagnosis: Invasive Ductal Carcinoma ER/PR -, Her2 +

Stage: 3a with additional diagnosis in November 2013 of same cancer on the skin of the same breast

Tip: I used essential oils a lot during my treatment. They helped tremendously with my neuropathy and side effects of chemotherapy. I loved using peppermint to settle my stomach and to get relief from headaches, and lavender to help me sleep.

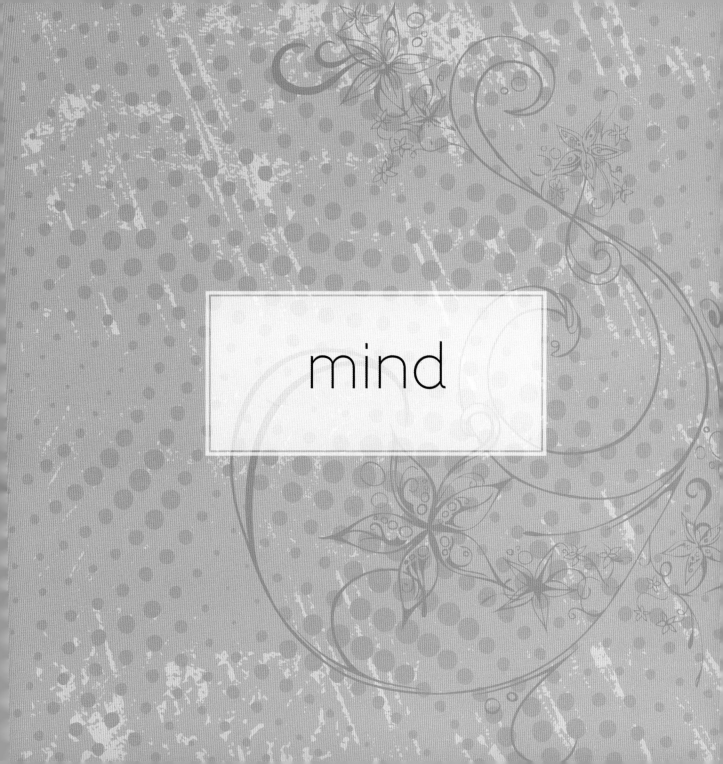

mind

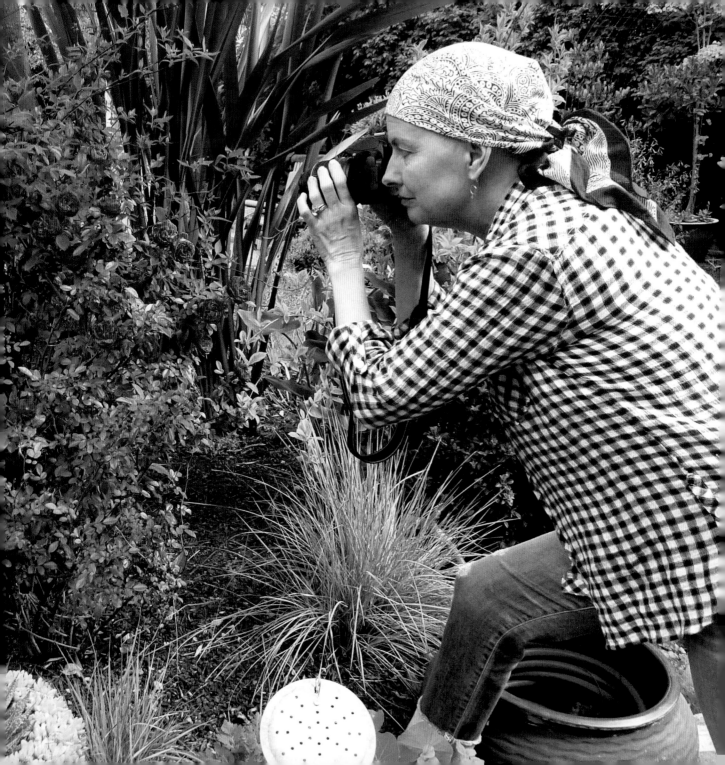

FIVE

Keep It Sharp

When your world is turned upside down and your medications and cancer treatment have a debilitating effect on your emotions and ability to function...it can be easy to give in. While we certainly will all have days where it's okay to simply say, "I just need to let myself feel sad or angry right now," the trick is not to stay in that place where your feelings get darker and your mind becomes more foggy. Allow your garden to heal your mind, keep it sharp, and ultimately bring you joy in the midst of the difficulties.

Planning & Visualizing Skills

There will be days, perhaps right after surgery or following each chemotherapy treatment, when you need bed rest. Or perhaps – unfortunately – you've experienced some side effects or complications to your treatment and are hospitalized. When you cannot do actual physical work in your garden, no worries – you are still a gardener! There are a number of activities that you can do to keep your brain engaged and to encourage forward thinking (particularly during a time when you might be fearing for your future).

CATALOGUES FOR INSPIRATION. Start with gathering up seed, plant and bulb catalogues to help you begin visualizing. In early spring every year, I am inundated with plant and seed catalogues in the mail; these are eye candy for the gardener, and you don't even have to order anything. I'm not much of a bulb gardener, but I recently received an entire catalogue on iris bulbs, and it kept me captivated for an entire evening. Look through the catalogues and earmark pages with products that look interesting to you so you can go back and order at the

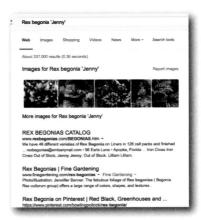

appropriate time for your area.

PLANT HUNTING. Go on a hunt for a particular type of plant that you've heard about but can't find – I love houseplants, Rex begonias in particular. I've heard that there is a 'Jenny' cultivar out there, and you can bet I spent some time trying to hunt it down. I haven't found it yet (I'm determined, though!) but just the process of following leads and doing Google searches has entertained me for hours.

PINTEREST. Another thing I love is Pinterest. For those of you who are not on this social site, it's literally a virtual bulletin board where you "pin" ideas for pretty much everything in your life. I currently have 51 boards with about 2800 pins, and my boards feature all types of categories, from gardening to recipes and interior décor. I have the Pinterest app on my iPad and have spent many hours "pinning" while recuperating from surgery

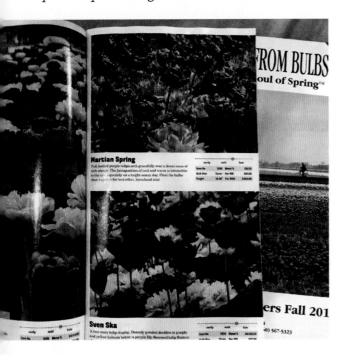

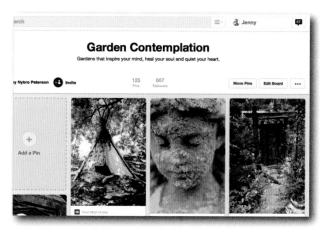

and treatment. Now that I think of it, the reason I bought my iPad in the first place was because I was spending so much time in waiting rooms and I didn't want to read old magazines while waiting to hear my name called. I brought my iPad with me to every chemo treatment and built up my Pinterest boards during that time. It was fun, interactive and helped me to plan ahead when actual gardening was off the table.

GARDEN MAGAZINES. These can be another source of inspiration while you're inside, and these days there is no shortage of publications for any garden activity you can think of. There are magazines for small space gardens, gardening in your particular state or region, garden design, cottage gardens, urban farms, houseplant

gardening, edible gardening and more. Keep a stack handy when you're down for the count — the inspiring photographs and informative articles will keep your brain humming right along.

GARDEN BOOKS. If you want to get more in-depth, don't forget your garden books! Now, I actually *wrote* my first book while going through treatment because it was the middle of summer in Texas and I was very sensitive to the heat. It was a perfect thing to do while my body was going through so much; my co-author and publisher were wonderful and supportive. Now, I'm not suggesting that you write a garden book (or any book), but reading them and gathering inspiration and ideas is a great idea during this time.

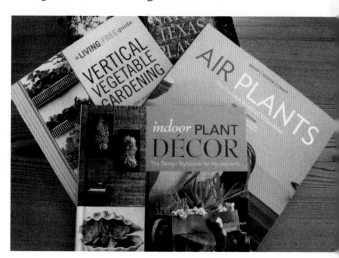

Measuring & Plotting

What to do when you've read everything and are just itching to put all that inspiration to good use? If you need a break from magazines, catalogues and books, but are still not ready to get out to physically garden, try plotting out a new garden bed. The physical act of drawing out and plotting new beds or garden features helps your brain to stay wired and logical; it's also helpful to do something mechanical like this when your emotions might be on overload. With just a few basic materials you can start to put your ideas on paper, so when your body catches up to your mind, you're ready to go.

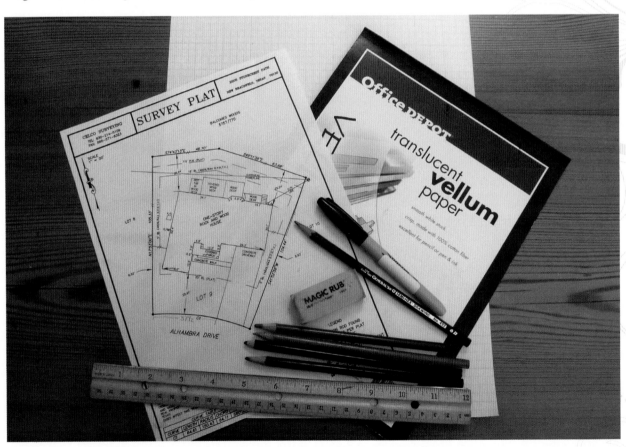

Materials

(all available at craft stores or even office supply stores)

- **Graph paper** – I like standard graph paper with ¼" grid marks.
- **Tracing paper or vellum** – Vellum is more translucent so it's easy to see the graph paper underneath.
- **A copy of your property's plot plan** (This is optional but helpful if you want your garden plan to be drawn to scale. The plot plan is usually found with your mortgage papers and includes all the dimensions of your property and house.)
- **Pencil and eraser**
- **Straight edge ruler**
- **Sharpie, optional**
- **Colored pencils, optional**

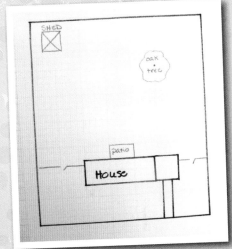

1. Slip a piece of graph paper underneath your tracing paper or vellum.

2. Using the graph paper underneath as your guide and your plot plan for measurements, draw the boundaries of your property according to a scale you have determined (for example, every ¼" square on your graph paper can equal 1 or 2 feet). Add your house with proper dimensions on your property.

3. Add in any other feature you might have (pool, shed, vegetable garden, etc.). These may or may not be scaled to their actual proportions, but it's more important to simply sketch in the proper location and relative size/shape.

4. Now have fun experimenting with new beds and features – a new mixed perennial border, a chicken coop, a deck extension or a fire pit area. Simply draw them in and spend some time figuring out the best locations for each feature and how to transition from one part of your garden to another.

I sometimes get fancier and use colored pencils to further illustrate new features – that way, I can tell at a glance what's new or planned for the future, what's already in place, and what is designated as a garden area or a physical structure.

If you can't locate your plot plan, no worries. I've done the simplest of sketches using the same materials listed above while just guessing at the scale or proportions. This activity isn't about being perfect or creating something to submit to your Homeowners Association, this is only for you. Treatment and even years of recovery from it can create a foggy brain and a lack of focus, so activities like these simply help to keep your brain functioning properly while you plan out your future garden.

Because I developed lymphedema after my treatment ended, I am still unable to do some basic garden chores (wheelbarrowing, hauling heavy items, shoveling, hoeing, etc.). Heavy lifting and jarring motions exacerbate this condition and make my left arm swell. So I'm often the one who plans out what should go where, while my fiancé, Brett, is the heavy lifter and digger. I do have days when I miss that physical exertion in my garden, but

I'm becoming more and more "okay" with my new normal. You will, too. I promise.

Problem Solving

Gardens and plants always present us with opportunities to grow and learn – there are new plants or different cultivars to discover, a pesky bug problem that you've never encountered before, or a strange looking disease that is wiping out your roses. While you're recuperating, put on your detective hat to figure out what the problem is. It may even have been a problem you had in last year's garden but you never had the time to investigate what was going on.

I love online research. As part of my job as a writer and author, I'm constantly

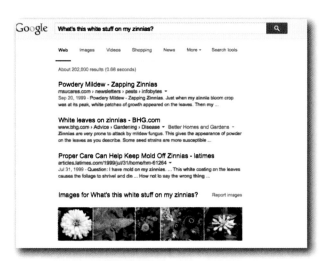

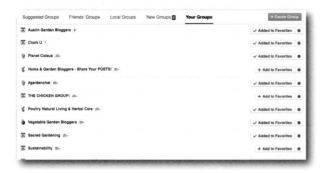

Googling plants, bugs, growth habits and the like, and I did it even more when I was housebound. I was also very lucky to have found some Facebook groups to participate in, from our Austin (Texas) area garden bloggers, to a general gardening group, to groups that focus on a particular plant like coleus or bamboo. I'm also a member of a Southwest Facebook garden group for people who live in our part of the United States. These groups afford the opportunity to commune and converse online with people who share your interests and can help you ID a plant, give advice about a pest or disease issue or applaud your garden success.

Your county extension office is another valuable resource – if you have a problem that you can describe on the phone, the Master Gardeners in the extension office are ready to help you. If you are well enough to drive to the office in person, bring clippings of plants with the pest or disease issue; they can help you figure out what's going on. Although I am not current with my certification, I was certified as a Master Gardener back in 2000, and I used to love helping people with their garden challenges.

Take Up Garden Photography

Photography is often an underutilized tool for visualization and creativity, and can be a valuable skill to have as a gardener. You don't need a fancy Nikon or Canon with detachable lenses (although those are wonderful) – just a simple point-and-shoot digital or even the camera on your

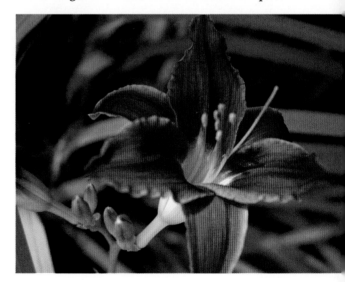

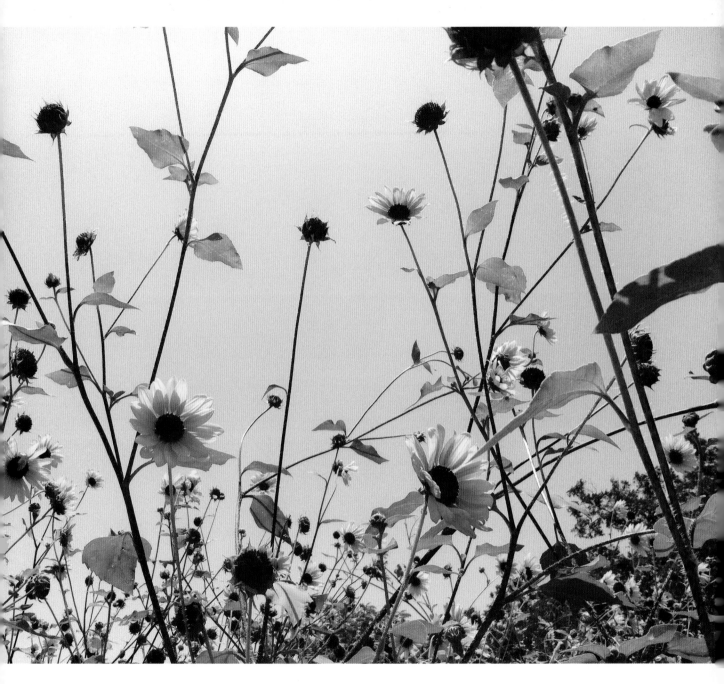

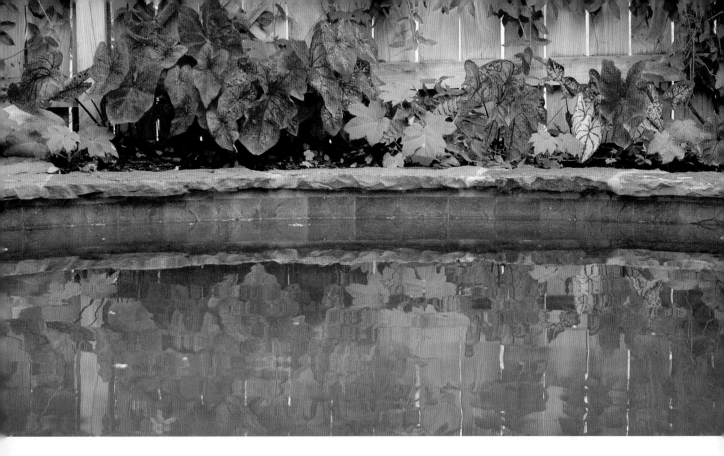

smartphone will do the trick. Photography is a way of getting out into the garden and participating in something artistic and creative while capturing an image that can bring you joy on a down day.

Practice taking shots of flowers or bugs close up, textures on leaves, sunlight through the foliage or your pets relaxing or playing in the garden. I've found that the best times for taking photographs is early in the morning or just at dusk – the sunlight is so much softer and can cast lovely shadows on your plants or other subjects. Overcast days are also great for photography, as well as days when there is a light mist. Avoid direct sunlight from the noon hour till the end of the afternoon; I'm usually not as pleased with the results at those times because the sun is simply too strong.

If you want to play around with your smartphone camera, there are many apps that make it easy to produce spectacular garden or nature shots. My two favorites right now are Camera+ and Over, but I've included a more extensive list in the sidebar. One of my favorite things to do is to put my camera on panoramic mode ("pano" on the iPhone), take a pic of a more expansive view, then add a filter in Camera+ and add text in Over. Because apps are ever-changing and evolving, please check your app store for the freshest photography app out there to begin experimenting. Many of them are free, so it won't cost you anything to try it. I do have some that cost up to about $4.00, but I figure that's a very low cost risk even if I don't like it.

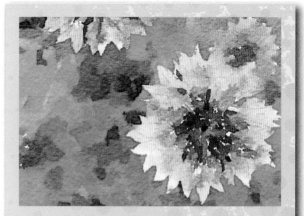

Smartphone Photography Apps

- **Camera+** (filters, color enhancing and adding frames)
- **Over** (adds words and artwork over your image)
- **Waterlogue** (transforms your images into watercolor "paintings")
- **Instacollage** (creates collages out of several images)
- **Photo Grid** (collage maker and special effects)
- **Simply Picture** (creates frames)
- **Reflection** (creates water reflections in images)
- **Pencil Sketch** (transforms images into pencil sketches)

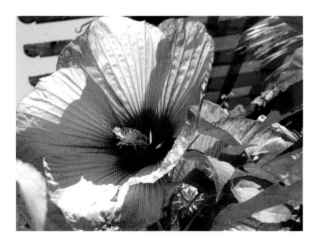

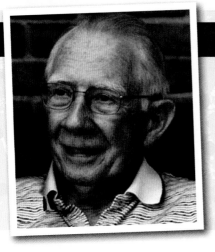

Survivor Spotlight

Name: Fred

Age at diagnosis: 70

Diagnosis: Malignant Melanoma

Stage: I don't remember but I had a recurrence 9 years later.

Tip: My wife is an avid gardener and I worked with her in the gardens as a way to keep busy and not think about the cancer. That helped her, of course, but it was also helping me.

Once you've taken the shots and edited them the way you want, share them online, email to friends and family or create a photo album (at home or online) to mark your experiences both as a gardener and as a photographer – you'll be surprised and delighted as you track your progress this way.

I hope that I am reminding you that gardening is so much more than planting and tending. Without all the planning and head-scratching time, nobody's garden would look great or thrive. Use this time in your recovery to tend to your garden in a different way – it will be there for you when your body is healed and ready to go. You are still "you," and you are still a gardener. ～

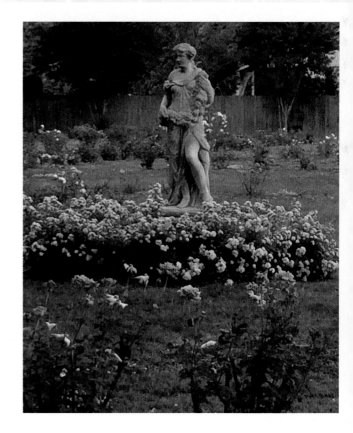

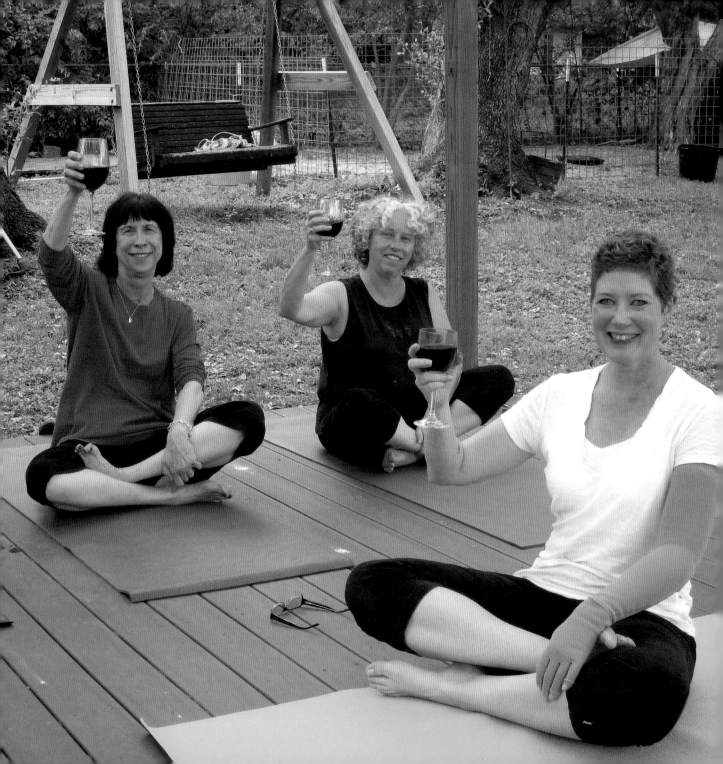

SIX

Build the Community

*L*et's face it – cancer can leave you feeling alone and isolated. You may not be able to do the things you once could, and you feel your world shrinking. You may not know how to reach out, and sometimes our friends and family, despite their best intentions, don't quite know what to say or do, so they say or do nothing. I told Brett during treatment, "I feel like people are trying their best to be supportive, but at the end of the day, that chemo IV is only going into *my* arm." It's okay to allow those feelings to surface, but I don't want any of you to stay in that place. Feeling isolated during treatment and recovery is a very dark place to be.

We've all experienced this, but there is no need for this to be your day-in and day-out reality. Of course, you will have your days when this is exactly how you feel, and while you may prefer to build memories with your friends and family around anything but cancer, cancer is a part of your life. How about letting your garden be a place to gather and build those memories, and to allow your plants and outdoor spaces to bring you together with the people who love and support you?

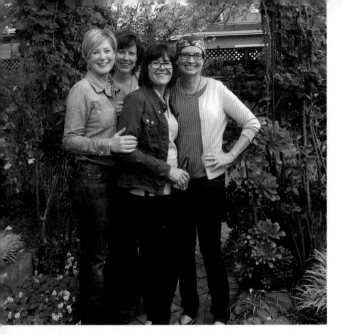

Enlist Help

You're in chemo and it's hot outside. Or, your hormones are doing the flip-flop and it's hot outside. Or, you just feel weak and it's hot (or cold) outside. The thing about the garden is that it doesn't stop doing its garden thing because you're not feeling well. The seasons come and go, weeds need pulling, seeds need sowing, plants need watering. The very last thing you want is for your garden to be neglected because you aren't feeling up to the task.

My father used to say, "What are friends for if you can't use them?" And I can't think of a better way to use them! Towards the middle of my treatment, I'd bought some vegetable transplants from the garden center, but I wasn't feeling well and hadn't gone out to plant them. And my Brett was working overtime to hold the fort down while I was ill, often coming home late in the day, exhausted. When I mentioned this to our dear friends Sherry and Jacque, who live across the street, they both exclaimed, "Why didn't you say anything? We'll be right over!"

They came right across the street and we walked out to the garden, wine glasses in hand. I showed them what I had and where I wanted them planted, and those two went to work. It didn't take long, and it wasn't difficult, but to have the two of them there to help me tend my garden was a priceless gift. I wish I'd taken a picture of that day, but I'm here to encourage you to 1) ask your friends and family for help, and 2) record it with 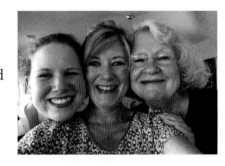 pictures, even if just on your phone's camera. These pictures will remind you, on down days, of who your Village is.

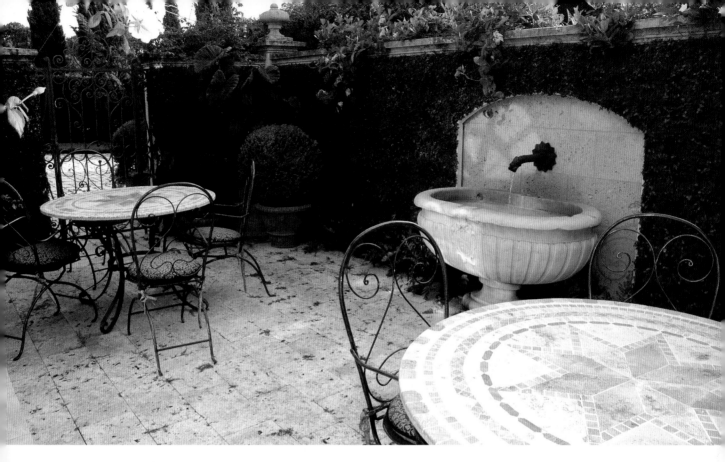

Create a Gathering Area

You might already have a gathering area in your garden, whether it's large or small. It could be a patio, a deck, a fire pit area or your pool. It will do your heart good during this time to make one of those places special. When family and friends stop by with dinner or just want to check on you, your garden can become a welcoming host.

This is more than simply creating an area that's pretty, and it doesn't have to be expensive and time-consuming. If you're not feeling well, the last thing I'd encourage you to do is to take on more than you need to. But creating these special spots for gathering and intimate talks is invaluable, as amazing conversation and healing moments can happen there. And I'm also not suggesting you do

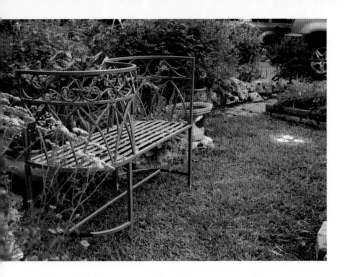

all of this yourself – if you get the urge to, do a quick reality check and see the previous section, "Enlist Help!"

- Have a bistro table and two chairs on your front porch or terrace.
- Put up a 2-person swing in the big oak tree with cozy pillows and a warm throw.
- Place chairs or flat-topped boulders around a movable fire pit for warmth.
- Throw an outdoor tablecloth over your picnic table or patio table and keep a vase of cut flowers from your garden in the center.
- Pull up a couple of chaise longues with a side table to relax with a friend.

- Set a garden bench in the yard or in the garden.
- If you have a more public side yard or front area where passersby walk, it could be fun to add seating out there as well so your neighbors can say a quick hello.

We had many times when our friends on the street would stop by for Happy Hour – it became something of a ritual every Friday night. Most times it would be on the front porch, but sometimes it was on our back patio or my newly-built yoga deck. We'd do a little yoga, laugh at how bad we were, and then have Bloody Marys. Please check with your doctor about drinking alcohol during your treatment – you might not feel like it anyway, but it's smart to get your oncologist's advice before imbibing. I liked

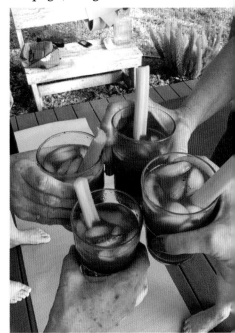

to have Happy Hour just that one night a week, and usually only one drink. It became something I really looked forward to because we all took turns making up a new cocktail recipe and the companionship and laughter were a balm for my soul.

Visit Gardens with Friends

As I neared the end of treatment, I started going out more and more and even took some business trips. I went to Ohio to work on our first book with my dear friend and co-author, Kylee, and then a number of us attended the Garden Writer's conference in Tucson the week I finished chemo.

"What?" you say, "You hopped on a plane the week you finished chemo? Are you insane?" Well, probably! But remember what I wrote in the intro to this book? My oncologist, Dr. Rubin de Celis, always encouraged me to live my life throughout treatment and particularly during recovery. He said, "Don't make your entire life about cancer; you can't live like that," and he was right. He told me that if I had any complications to go to the ER – and yes, I had some complications, and yes, I went to the ER. But it would've happened at home, too, and at least I had my friends around me to build fantastic memories.

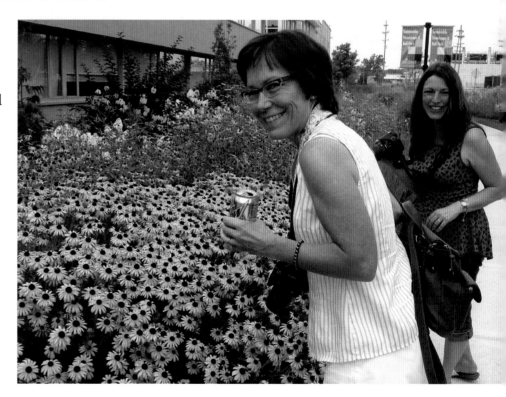

So, check with your doctor first, and then grab a friend or two and visit:

- Botanical gardens
- Show gardens
- Private garden tours
- Trial or test gardens
- Another friend's garden
- Wildflower centers
- National parks

Invite Your Club Over

Are you a member of a garden club, but haven't felt well enough to attend? Or perhaps you are hesitant to go out after losing your hair, or need to stay close to home because of your side effects? As you acclimate to a slower pace for a while, invite your club to meet at your house and in your garden. Don't make a big deal of it – even if your particular club likes to pull out all the stops for their meetings. Arrange ahead of time to have the other members organize it and bring refreshments; just enjoy the company of people who have been a regular part of your life and routine around a hobby that you all love.

Some garden clubs like to dress up for their meetings; this is particularly true in the South, I'm told. I remember when I was going through chemotherapy and I

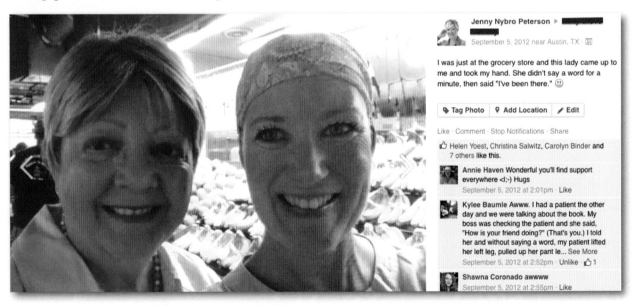

Jenny Nybro Peterson ▶
September 5, 2012 near Austin, TX

I was just at the grocery store and this lady came up to me and took my hand. She didn't say a word for a minute, then said "I've been there." 🙂

🏷 Tag Photo   📍 Add Location   ✏ Edit

Like · Comment · Stop Notifications · Share

👍 Helen Yoest, Christina Salwitz, Carolyn Binder and 7 others like this.

Annie Haven Wonderful you'll find support everywhere <J;-) Hugs
September 5, 2012 at 2:01pm · Like

Kylee Baumle Awww. I had a patient the other day and we were talking about the book. My boss was checking the patient and she said, "How is your friend doing?" (That's you.) I told her and without saying a word, my patient lifted her left leg, pulled up her pant le... See More
September 5, 2012 at 2:52pm · Unlike · 👍 1

Shawna Coronado awwww
September 5, 2012 at 2:55pm · Like

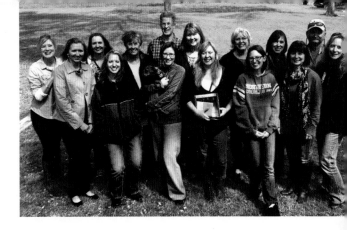

was self-conscious about wearing my new wig, Brett said to me one day, "Honey, why don't you get yourself dressed up and I'll take you out to lunch?" It was the best thing for my sense of self to put on a little makeup, slip into something that didn't resemble pajamas or yoga pants, and go out with my beloved. We weren't out that long because I tired easily at that time, but I recall it so fondly because Brett understood that I wasn't feeling attractive or normal and wanted to help.

I say this because for a few hours, if you can muster the energy when your club comes over, it's worth it to get a little dressed up. Ladies, put on a sundress and gentlemen, don a fresh shirt — sometimes the exterior has a way of influencing the way you feel on the inside.

Have a Seed & Plant Sharing Party

I belong to an Austin-area garden blogging group. It's a group of about 55 of us who blog about gardening – some of us are professionals, but we are all simply passionate about gardening and blogging about it. We have a monthly get-together called a "Go-Go" (I'm not sure I remember how that name came to be!) where we gather at a different member's garden and help him or her out with a problem part of their outdoor space. This isn't a work day; we're simply throwing out ideas and sometimes we even draw them out on paper. There are usually people who bring transplants of daylilies or agave pups to share, and there's usually food and drink involved. It's very casual and fun.

Because I often work on Saturdays when the Go-Go's take place, I can't always attend the gatherings. But I can tell you that I went to several while I was going through treatment, and it made me feel involved and, well, normal. It's not the same as a garden group, but the camaraderie is priceless.

If you have a group like this, invite them over – this is the easiest group to have in your garden because it's so much more laid back than a formal club. And if you don't have a club like mine, simply invite some of your garden friends. Whip up some iced tea or ice water with lemon slices and call it good – then enjoy the company of friends while you trade seeds, swap divisions and pups, and get advice on what's eating your okra. If you have some plants that need to be divided, tell your comrades ahead of time and they can do it for you. I'm sure they'd be pleased to, because not only are they helping you, they get to share in the bounty!

There's a saying that gardeners are the most generous people, and I've found that to be true. They also tend to be very "grounded" and relaxed people, just what you need at a time like this.

Let Your Garden Host Your Head Shaving

When I was about ready to shave my hair, I'd already cut off about 18". I had decided before my first chemo appointment that I really didn't want to have over a foot and a half of long hair to simply fall out, so I would do it in stages. I first cut it to a very short, almost pixie

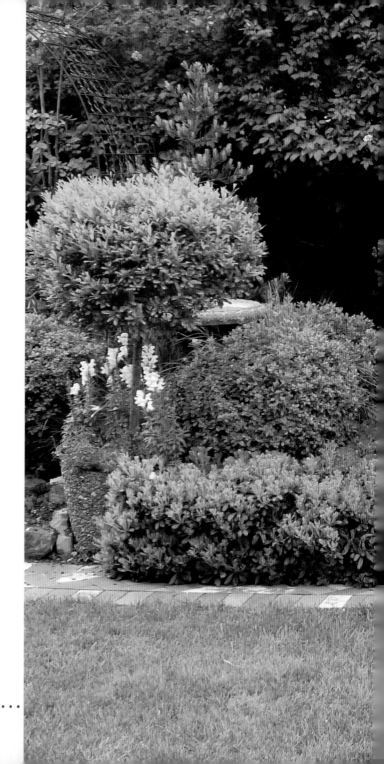

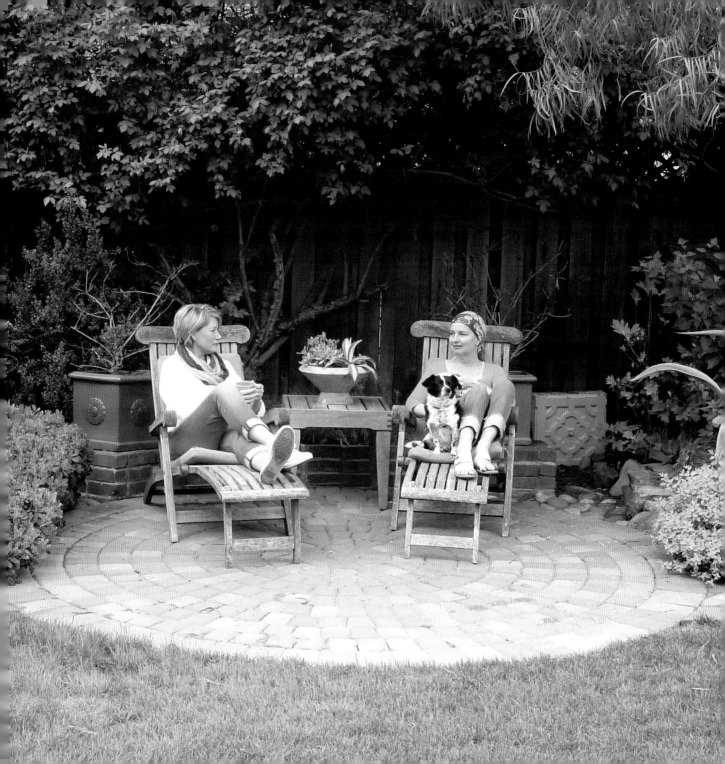

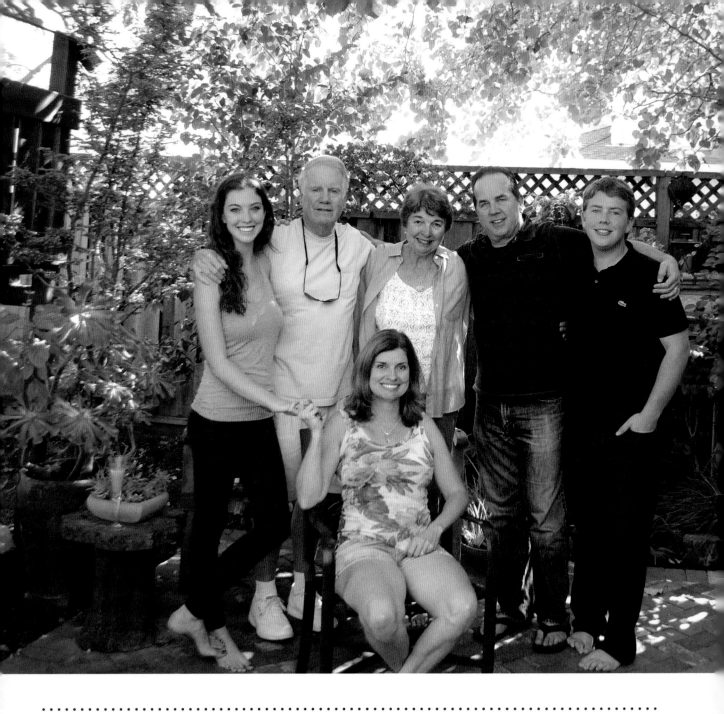

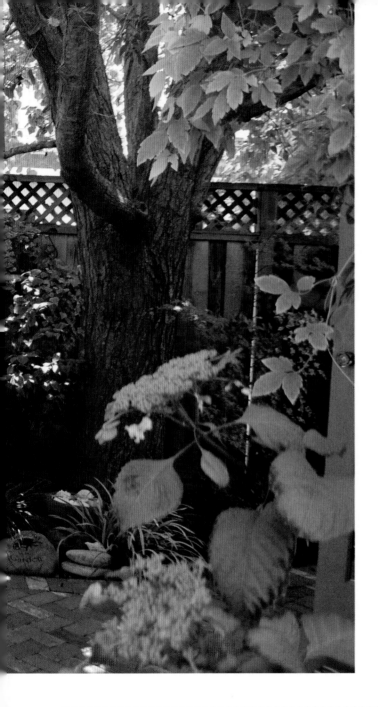

cut. Then, a week after chemo, my family gathered at my sister-in-law Turid's hair salon after hours, and her stylist shaved my hair down to a #2 buzz cut. We had wine and took pictures and laughed – it felt good to be taking some control with my family there to cheer me on. It was a powerful evening.

My friend Rebecca did it differently. She has been known for her thick hair that she styled into a flip – it was almost an iconic look for her, actually. And when she was diagnosed with breast cancer, she took the head shaving party (I use that word loosely) out to her garden. Now, Rebecca has the most gorgeous garden I've almost ever seen (she's a landscape designer and has lived in that house for many years), and when she wrote a blog post about her experience, I thought it was perfect for her.

She invited her family and a couple of friends into her beautiful back yard garden. Then she sectioned off her hair by tying hair bands around it, like ponytails all over her head. Then, each member of her immediate family cut off one of the ponytails – helping them to feel emotionally connected to the process – before her friend's stylist neatened it up with a razor.

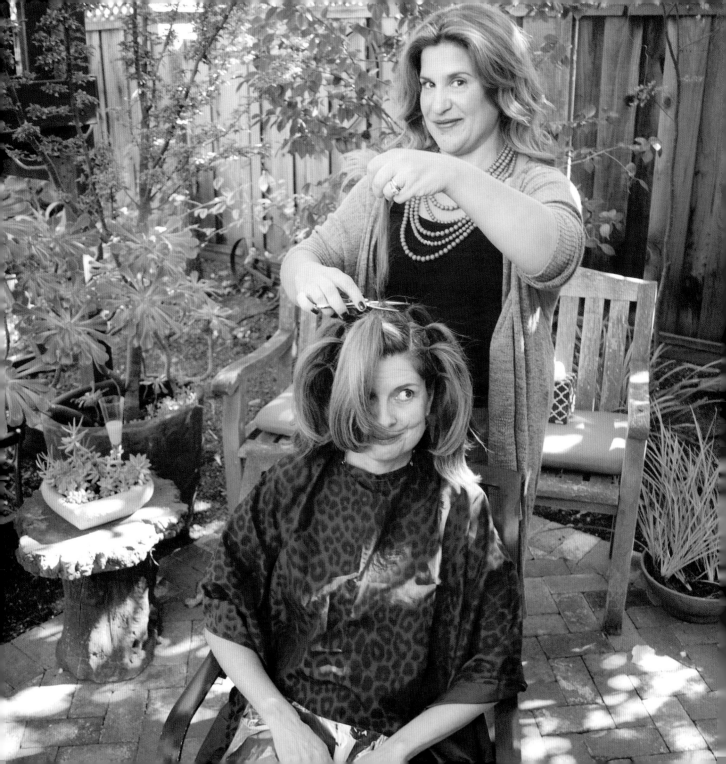

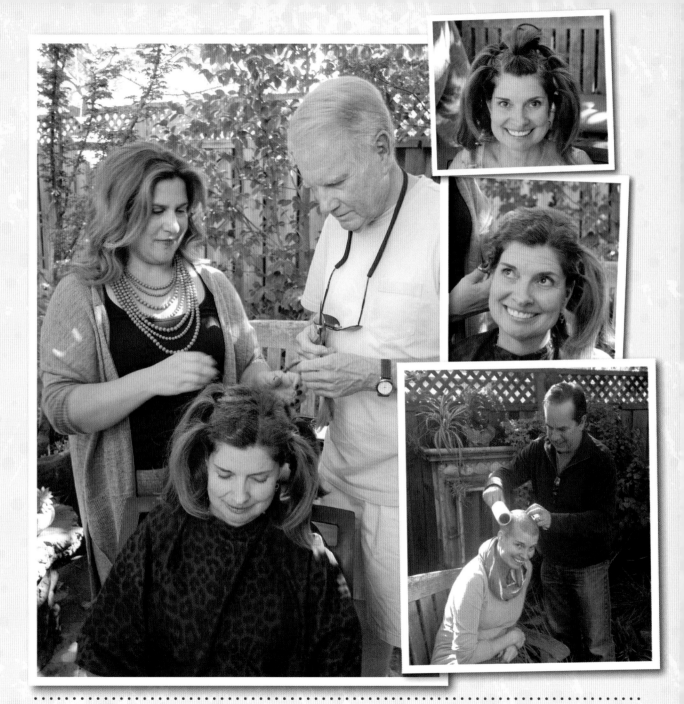

"During the entire hour it took to shave my head, I felt my garden's tender embrace as I underwent this transformation. Along with my family holding my hands and surrounding me with their love, my garden was there, helping to usher me forward."

~ Rebecca Sweet

Rebecca donated her hair to Locks of Love, and she says that one of her favorite photographs was when she and her husband, Tom, returned to the garden a week later to lint-roller off the stubble that was beginning to fall out. Even though it's highly emotional, sometimes the humor of the situation can be just what you need to lighten the mood. A lint roller? That's hilarious.

Whether you are a man or a woman, with long hair or short hair, the totally bald look is one instant indicator that you are going though cancer treatment. It may not be as noticeable on the gentlemen, but men still struggle with the head shaving after chemo. What a beautiful, poignant ritual to take this step in your garden, a place of warmth and intimacy for you and your loved ones. ∾

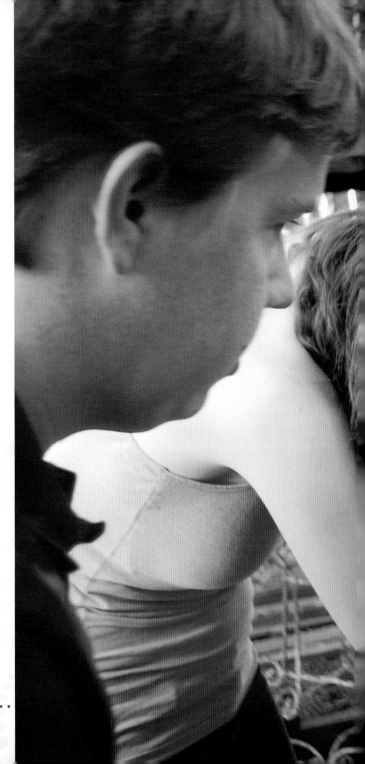

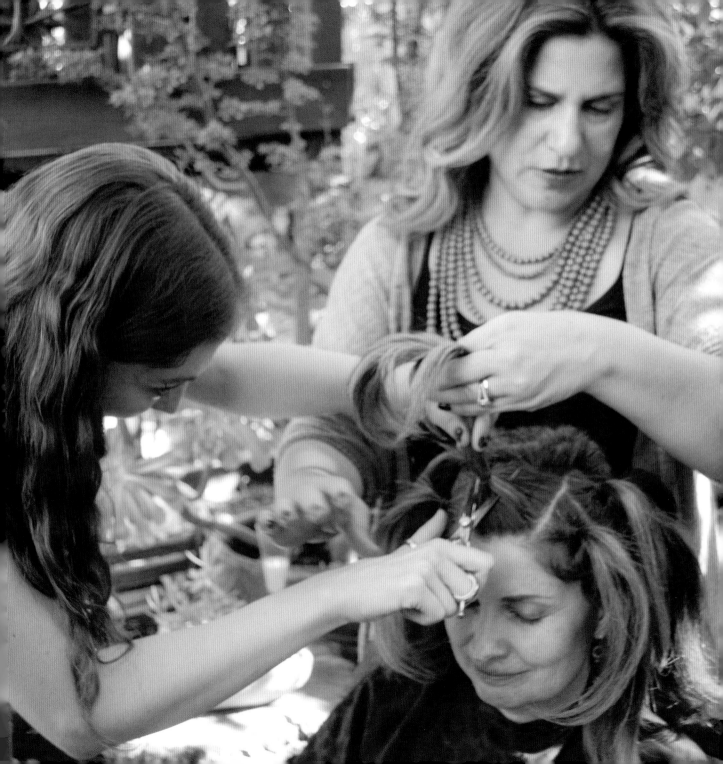

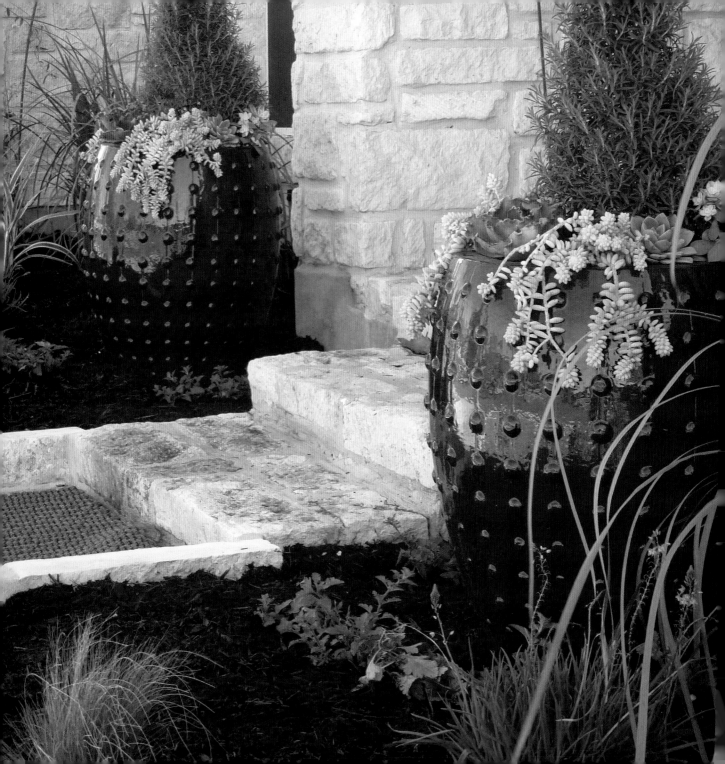

SEVEN

The Moody Blues

Anyone who's gone through a cancer diagnosis knows the emotional struggles that often go along with it. You're sad, frightened, angry, anxious, depressed, listless – perhaps not every day, but often enough to feel unbalanced and unsure of what to expect. Cancer can create feelings that you may have never experienced before, and those feelings can remain long after your treatment has ended. When I finished chemotherapy and radiation, my hair began to grow back in and people commented on how healthy I looked – yet I felt more sad and aimless than ever. And then I felt guilty. One person actually said to me, "You should feel thankful, not sad, that you are done with treatment and are alive."

Well, of course I was thankful, but that comment spurred very angry feelings in me. Cancer is not like having the flu for a few weeks. So my advice to you is to acknowledge the feelings you have without feeling guilty for having them, and do what you can to work your feelings out as you heal. One way to do this is by gardening – plants and gardens are proven blues busters, and they are timely reminders of how life continues on despite what we are going through.

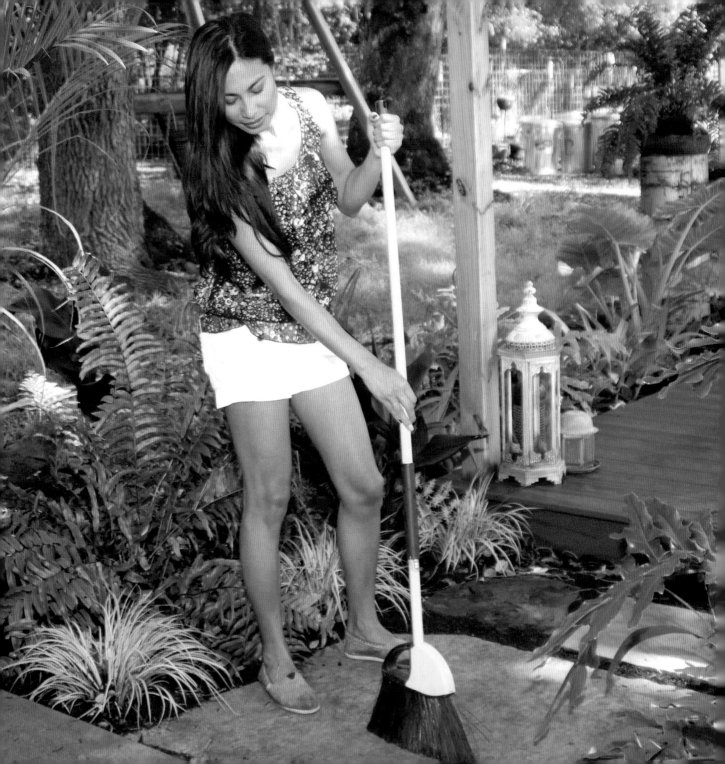

Match the Chore to the Mood

Not all garden chores are created equal. Some require more physical strength while others call for more thoughtfulness and finesse. When your feelings seem overwhelming and bordering on out of control, take it out to the garden and match the garden chore to the mood you are having. It's one of the most wonderful things about gardening – it's always there for you and will accept whatever chore you need to do. No judgment and no criticism here – your okra won't care if you're ugly crying with mascara running down your face, and the roses won't even notice that your clothes look like you got dressed in the dark. They're just glad you're out there.

Angry	Dig holes, weed with your hoe
Sad	Plant cheerful flowers in your favorite color
Introspective	Hand weed, water, sweep
Anxious	Trim, prune
Hopeless	Sow seeds, plant transplants
Thankful	Harvest

Let Your Garden Decide

I've been in such a state that I couldn't make the most simple of decisions, and I bet you've been there, too. Life seemed so overwhelming that just the thought of taking care of the garden and figuring out what needed to be done created feelings of dread in me – yet the thought of having my garden die from neglect was even more dreadful. During these times, just put on your garden shoes and move outside. Don't plan a damn thing, just go. Move. Breathe. Your garden will tell you what it needs.

You might even walk around crying – believe me, I've done it. A year after I finished treatment, I had some sudden and seemingly inexplicable side effects from my medications. Many post-treatment medications can create emotional instability, depression and even suicidal thoughts, and the meds that I took for chemo-induced nerve damage suddenly made me very unstable. For about 24 hours I was a basket case. I was inconsolable, wept constantly, felt totally hopeless and helpless. Not able to stand lying in bed a minute longer, I got up at 2 a.m. and wandered outside, crying. I walked

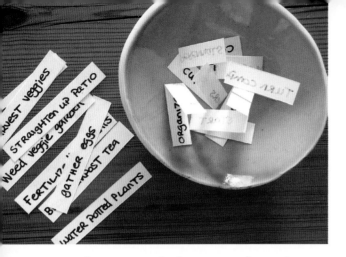

around my yoga deck, sat on the swing dangling my feet, listened to the occasional rooster crow from the chicken coop, all the while sobbing. It wasn't at all funny at the time, but I've since said that the only thing more dramatic would have been if there was a ghostly fog while I wandered around in a long white nightgown, à la Wuthering Heights.

That night was the most terrifying of my life, because I couldn't see how I would even want to live a minute more with the feelings I was having. But being outside, breathing in the night air, tuning in to the whispering sounds of the wind through the trees, feeling the ground underneath my feet – all of these things gently coaxed me out and beyond my immediate troubles. My garden, even in the shadows of night, created a sense of sanctuary and

enclosure for me, soothing my mind and my heart. Later, I created a bowl with garden chores written on scraps of paper, determined to be prepared should these feelings overtake me again. I wouldn't have to decide anything, I'd just pick a piece of paper and go outside and move.

During your darkest times, focus on breathing and just being – and what better place to do both than outside in your garden? Making the choice to go outside, even for a few minutes, and breathing in fresh air as you walk around can be just what you need to ease your difficult feelings.

Bring Music to the Garden

Music has long been known to control stress, reduce pain and improve brain function, so take it out to the garden with you. If you have a smartphone, tablet or iPod, you can create playlists of your favorite songs to get you going. If you don't have any of these gadgets, then simply take an old radio out with you and tune in to one of your favorite stations. The music you listen to can become the backdrop to your garden chores, giving added energy and meaning to what you are doing.

You can create playlists depending upon the mood you are in, but be careful that your playlist of sad songs doesn't keep you stuck in that down space. I like to mix up different music genres, tempos and moods with my playlists – listening to a funny yet thought-provoking John Prine song right after a deeply moving choral piece. It reminds me that, while life can be a struggle sometimes, something comical can happen in the midst of it, creating a healthy balance of the profound and ridiculous.

If you're struggling with depression, try creating an upbeat playlist to counter your feelings. It needn't be a sickeningly sweet mix of peachy keen songs ("I'm Walking on Sunshine," for example), but perhaps some upbeat tempos, uplifting lyrics or something you can dance to or sing along with is just what you need. As I was recovering, I'd go out to my chicken coop every morning to let the chickens out, and I found myself singing

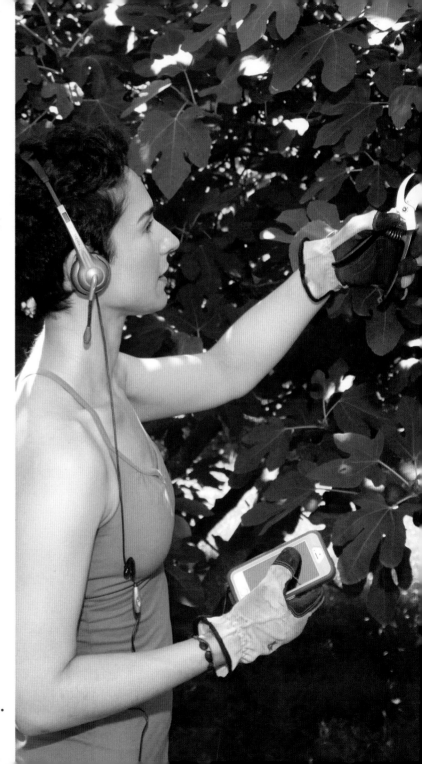

Beyonce's song "All The Single Ladies" to the hens (this was before we had roosters), dancing around as I threw down the chicken scratch, and I would start to laugh every time. Look for moments like these in your garden to cut loose and be a little silly, with music leading the way – it's seemingly small actions like these that keep you balanced.

Garden-Themed Playlist

- *Here Comes the Sun* by The Beatles
- *The Four Seasons* by Antonio Vivaldi
- *Summertime* by Ella Fitzgerald
- *Flower Child* by Lenny Kravitz
- *In the Garden* by Susan Tedeschi
- *It's a Big Old Goofy World* by John Prine
- *Jardin* by Gustavo Santaolalla
- *Let It Be* by The Beatles
- *Turn the Dirt Over* by Sea Wolf
- *Scarborough Fair* by Simon & Garfunkle
- *Build Me Up Buttercup* by The Foundations
- *Somewhere Over the Rainbow* by Israel "IZ" Kamakawiwo'ole

Develop a New Garden Hobby

When you learn something new, it's exciting because it gives you something to look forward to, and nobody is as passionate about something as a new convert is. So pick up a new hobby in the garden – start bird watching, learn vegetable gardening if you've only focused on ornamentals, grow roses, create a koi fish pond, or learn the botanical Latin name of every plant in your garden. When I finished treatment, we added chickens to our backyard, and while my fiancé had to do the coop cleaning chores as my immune system healed, taking care of the baby chicks, naming them and learning about their care lifted my spirits every day.

Choose a new garden hobby that aligns with your budget and energy – some are

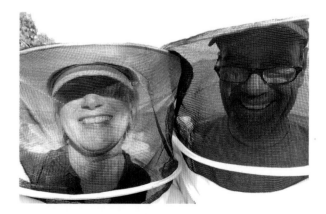

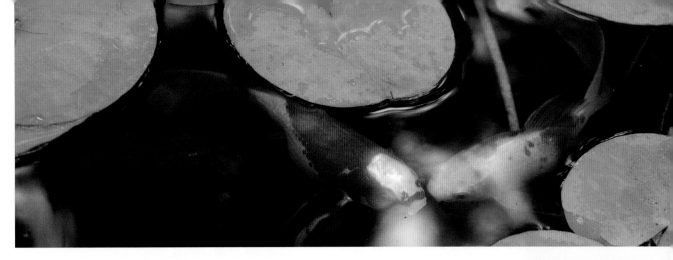

free and relatively simple to take up, while others require more start-up funds and attention. I recommend settling on only one new hobby, as your energy and focus may ebb and flow for a while, and starting too many new things can quickly become overwhelming. Let this new interest be something that you've always wanted to do, something that nourishes you and builds some anticipation in your life when other things seem so uncertain. As I healed, we also began making plans to add beekeeping to our backyard farm, so we enrolled in a class to learn the basics. We had a great time donning the protective gear and learning all the details with other bee enthusiasts, and it's given both of us another outdoor activity to look forward to.

In an odd kind of way, I was thankful for some of the "down time" that I had during treatment and recovery, as it allowed me to take time for myself to learn my new chicken-raising hobby. You might be a 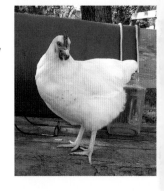 lot like me in that I sometimes feel guilty for taking time off or doing things that are simply fun, but while you're going through treatment you have a built-in pass to focus on yourself and getting healthy, so take advantage of this! You're not being lazy or unproductive – there is no harder work than recovering from cancer treatment and taking your bodily, emotional and spiritual health seriously.

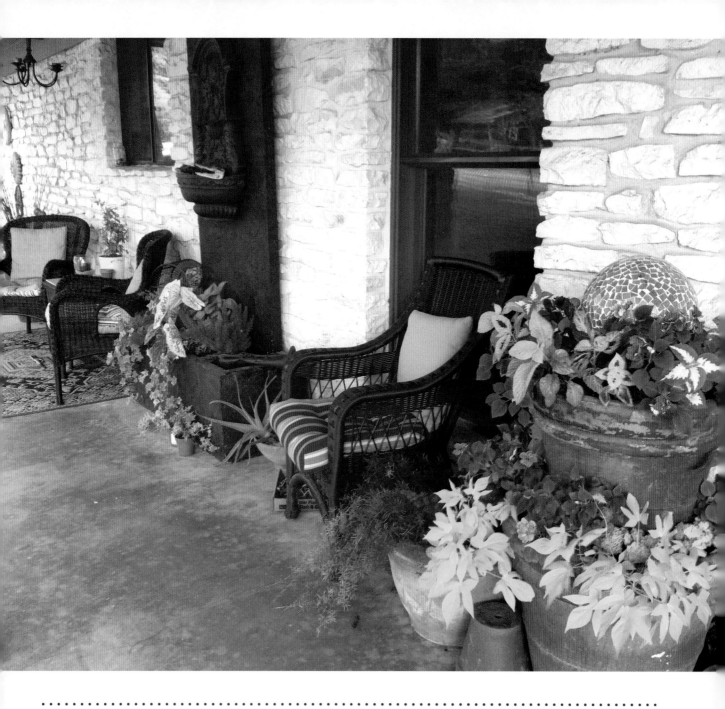

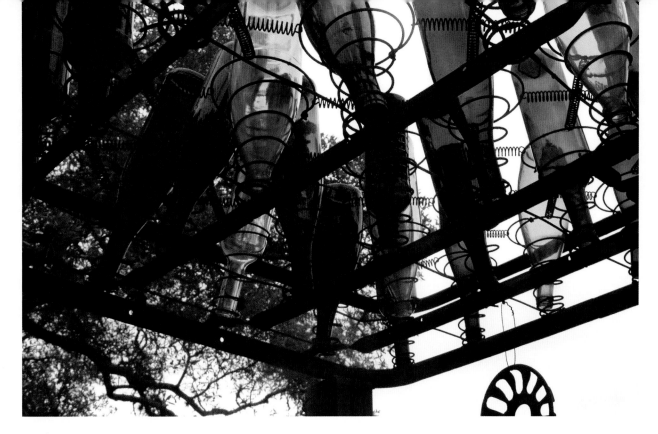

Focus on Just One Thing

In July of 2012, I had a lumpectomy followed up by a lymph node dissection. The second surgery was by far the more difficult, and left me feeling weak and overwhelmed – my range of motion was so severely impacted that for a time I needed help simply brushing my hair (this was before I lost all of my hair to chemo). Then I looked out into my yard every day, seeing only all the things that were left undone. I decided that while I couldn't rebuild the vegetable garden as I'd previously planned, I could tend to my houseplants and my front porch. My beautiful front porch became the scene of neighborhood happy hours every Friday evening. While the rest of my yard looked like hell, my porch became the center of my gardening life. I just had to let the other things go and focus on just one thing.

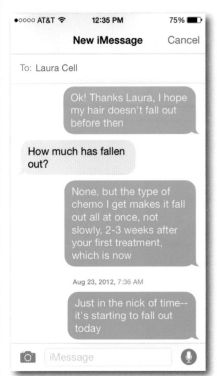

What is your "just one thing" while you are either going through treatment or recovering? Make it something that gives you real joy, as well as something that is the most important to you – for me, I decided that I could live with an ugly, dilapidated vegetable garden (it was functional, after all), but that it was very important to me to have a beautiful place where my friends and family and I could gather and relax. It not only relieved pressure to have everything looking great, it gave me great pleasure to create. When I made the decision to simply focus on my front porch, Brett and I made it fun – we invited our friends from across the street over and together we rearranged furniture, hung bird houses, placed a fountain and created two different seating areas. When we were done, we all sat down with cocktails to enjoy the new and beautiful gathering space that we'd created.

While I was writing this book, several cancer survivors sent me images of the "one thing" that they created as they were either going through treatment or healing from it. Patti (featured in one of my "Survivor Spotlights") emailed me that she was not a big gardener before her breast cancer diagnosis, but afterwards, she created a garden with pink geraniums in the shape of a ribbon. It became her labor of love that she tends to this day. Another gardener, Elayne, built an arbor with an old bedspring and bottles to channel her energy upwards as she and her husband struggled with cancer (photo on p.101).

As you feel able, consider creating something special like these gardeners did to remind yourself of what you'd like your focus to be, or to simply honor your own journey. It's a daily visual reminder of what you've come through.

REACH OUT. If even your "just one thing" is too overwhelming to start, please ask for help. With my range of motion issues, I wouldn't have been able to rearrange the porch furniture on my own,

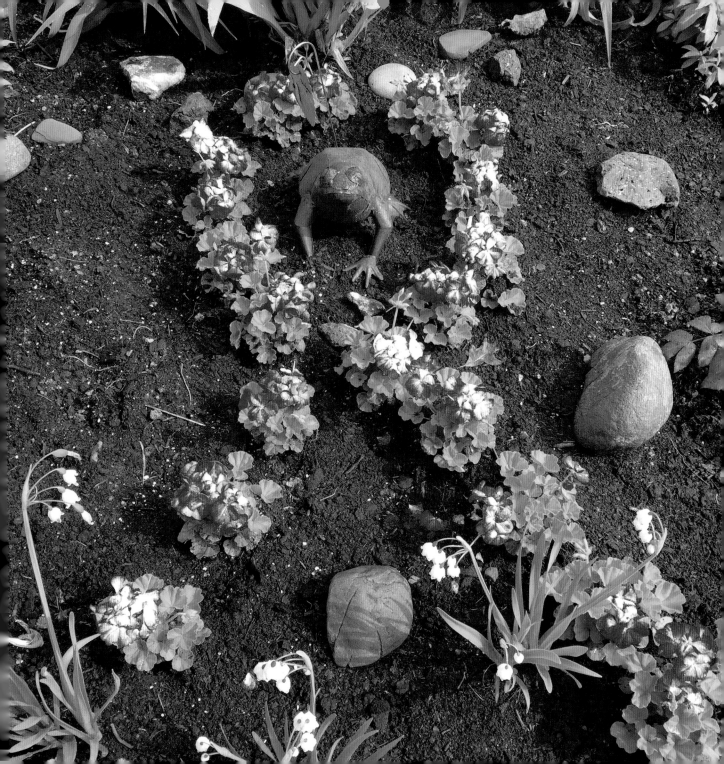

and while Brett could have done it by himself, that may have seemed to be "one more thing" to add to his already heavy load. Plus, our friends Sherry and Jacque really wanted to do something concrete to help, and they are gardeners as well – so it was a win-win for everyone. Once the front porch was in place, my job every day was to water the plants, keep the furniture clean and gently sweep leaves off the floor. It became something I really looked forward to, and our neighbors and passersby appreciated the beauty we'd created.

As you begin to heal more, go back to your "just one thing" list and add in another "just one thing" to your gardening routine. You may find that every couple of months you're adding in one more activity, but please honor your recovery by postponing activities that your body, mind or spirit is not ready for. Believe me, I felt a little silly on occasion saying out loud, "I'm not ready to lift that mulch bag yet," when I used to haul them around as if I was a pack mule – but you are not doing yourself any favors by pushing your recovery past where it needs to be at this moment, even if it looks to the world that you are 100% recovered.

"Just One Things"

- Houseplants
- Front entryway garden
- Front porch
- Back porch/patio/deck
- Window box
- Water feature
- Container plants
- Herb garden
- Vegetable garden

Take your immune system, muscular strength, lymphedema issues, scar tissue and healing incisions all into account as you slowly work your way back to a more regular routine.

Two years later, my vegetable garden is still ugly and dilapidated (see opposite). And that's okay – my garden taught me during treatment that life is all about priorities, accepting the ugly while creating the beauty. It's this always-changing contrast in the world around us that helps us to create both balance and a sense of peace – things that are very important to me in general, but particularly when I was going through recovery.

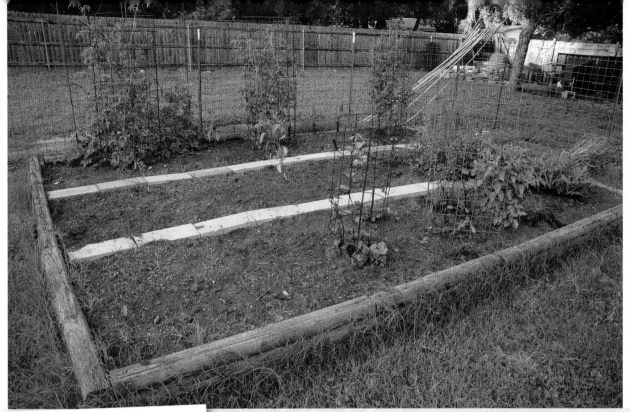

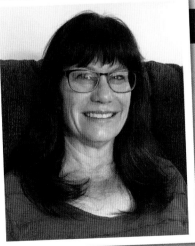

Survivor Spotlight

Name: Patti

Age at diagnosis: 55

Diagnosis: Breast & Thyroid Cancer at the same time

Stage: 0

Tip: Needing only a mastectomy with no radiation, I felt I had to remind women to take care of themselves. That same spring, I knew I needed a pink garden with a ribbon of pink geraniums center stage. I have brown thumbs but this garden has been a labor of love for me for the past three years. *(See Patti's pink garden on page 103.)*

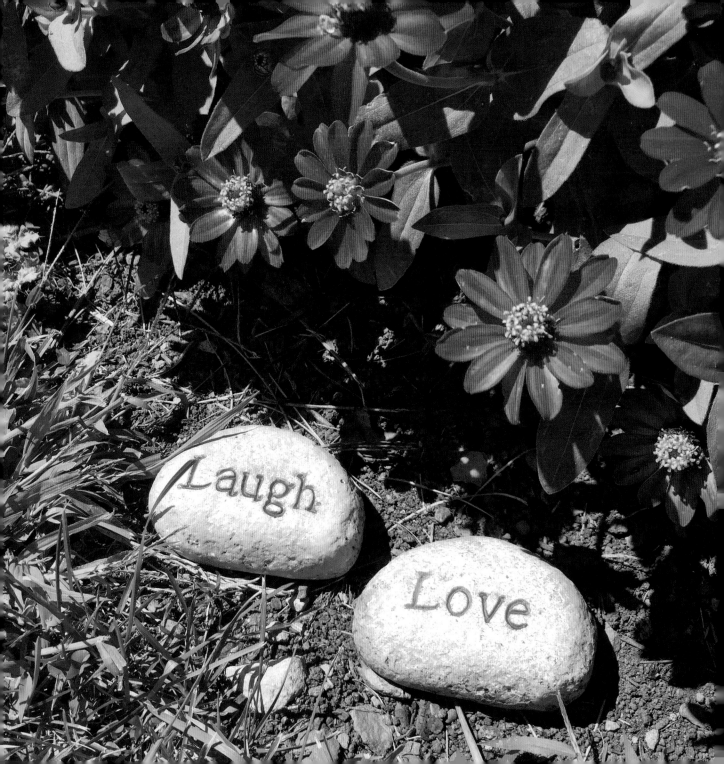

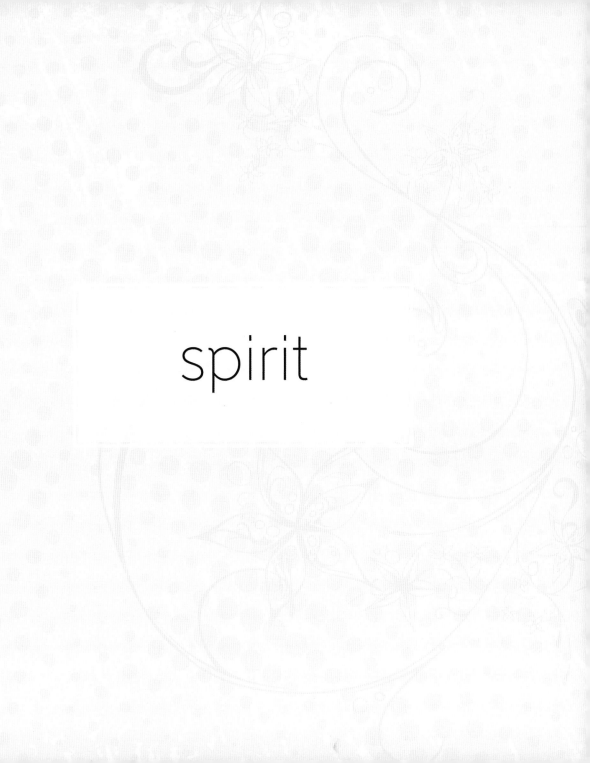

spirit

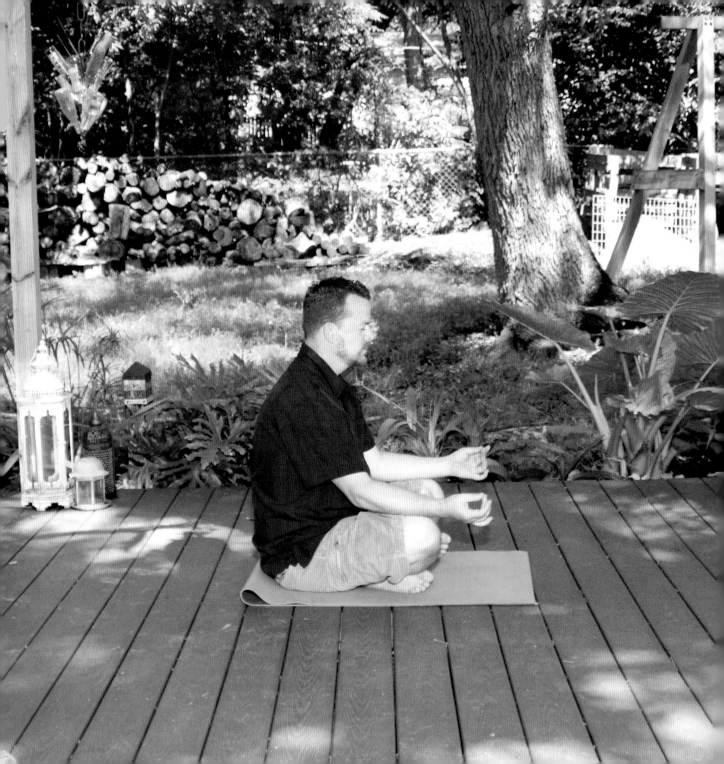

EIGHT

Connect with Spirit

When you feel alone, afraid, despairing, angry – all of these things and more – how do you connect with Spirit? With God? With the Universe? Maybe you don't have the words, as your grief may be too deep, or perhaps you have never had an experience of anything overtly spiritual before and aren't sure what to "do." Relax. Our previous chapters have dealt with things to do; now we're going to focus on simply being and connecting. Your expression of this does not need to follow a book right now, and it doesn't need to look like your neighbor's. Whatever you are seeking, the garden can show you and reveal to you.

Prayer & Meditation

While prayer and meditation can be overtly religious, it is really simply a way of communicating with the Creator or the Universe. In prayer, you can ask for things you need such as peace, healing, comfort or help for your loved ones, while in meditation you can sit quietly and let your heart receive what it will. There is no judgment here; if you have a thought, just be aware of it and then let it go.

I've found that my garden is the perfect place for me to pray and meditate – certainly, I have other places indoors where I do these things (particularly in inclement weather), but my garden invites

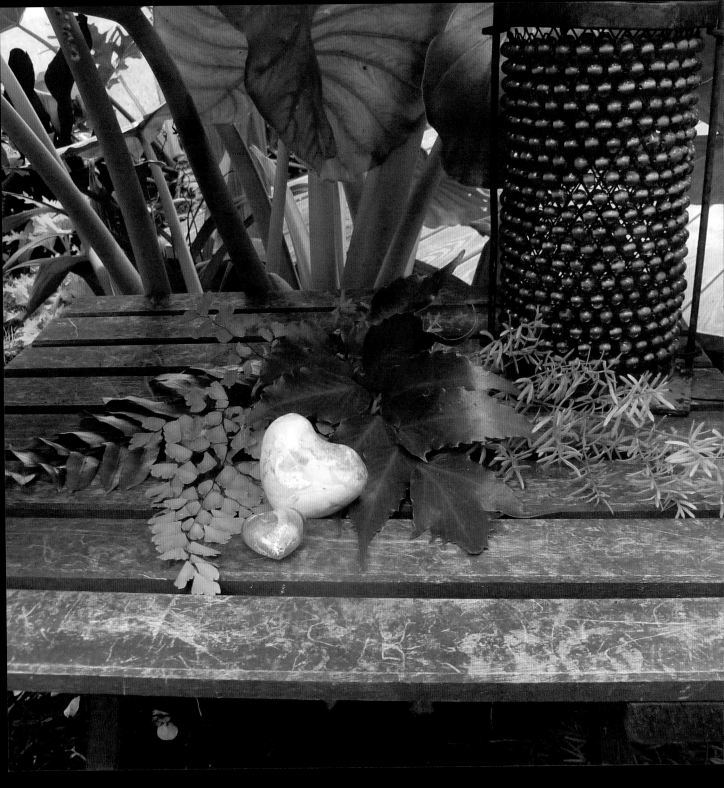

my body to relax in a way that I can't quite duplicate indoors. The warm sunshine, the birds chirping, the cool breeze and the sounds of my neighborhood all work together to melt the knots out of my muscles, and when my body is relaxed, my heart and mind follow.

In the places of the garden where you like to pray or meditate, consider choosing plants that have traditional meanings to serve as living reminders to you of what you are seeking. You can invite friends and family to a garden party where they each bring a plant or a flower with the meaning they would like to contribute as well – I've often thought of inviting my breast cancer survivor friends over to do just that. In the years since we've all been diagnosed, we've celebrated clear scans, high-fived hair growing back in, cherished pregnancies we thought would never happen, and grieved our friends who have died. Such a garden would be a beautiful and poignant show of love and community.

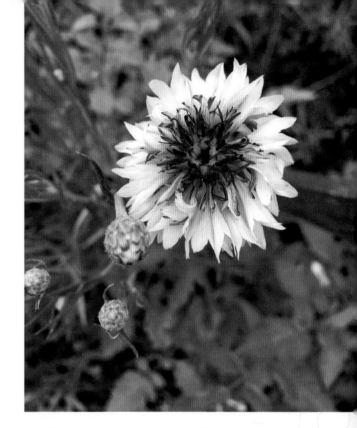

The Language of Flowers

There is a language, little known,
Lovers claim it as their own.
Its symbols smile upon the land,
Wrought by nature's wondrous hand;
And in their silent beauty speak,
Of life and joy, to those who seek
For Love Divine and sunny hours
In the language of the flowers.

–The Language of Flowers, London, 1875

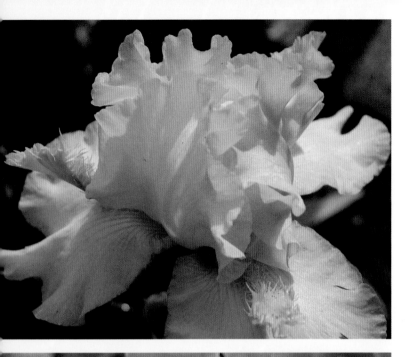

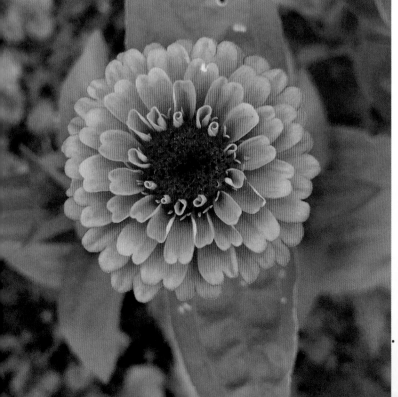

What Plants Mean

Coneflower: strength, health
Daisy: innocence, hope
Dill: luck
Esperanza: hope
Fern: sincerity
Foxglove: protection
Goldenrod: encouragement
Iris: faith, hope
Lavender: longevity
Peony: healing
Poppy (red): consolation
Rosemary: remembrance
Rue: grace, clear vision
Sage: wisdom
Sweet pea: courage
Thyme: courage, strength
Verbena: peace
Zinnia: thoughts of absent friends

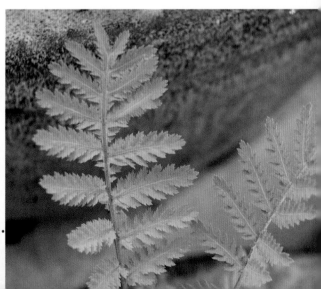

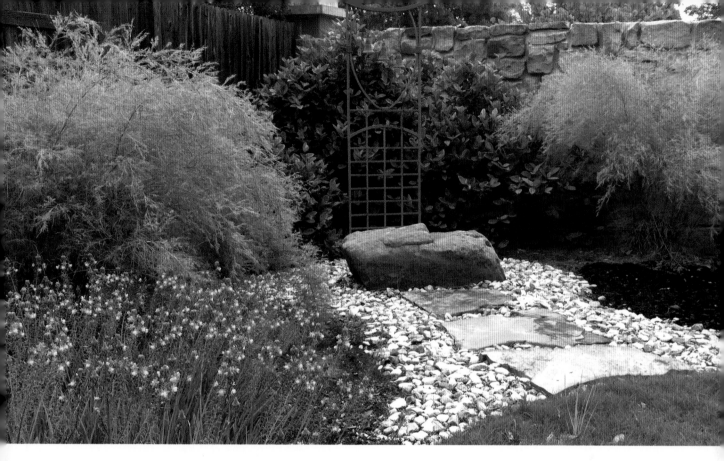

You can also simply use plants that evoke a particular feeling to you. In my yoga deck garden, I've used plants that are very lush and tropical looking – elephant ears, canna, philodendron, coleus, ferns...which seems peculiar to me since I don't actually prefer the tropics or the beach. But these plants say "relax" to me; they are soft and enclosing, with their hint of rainforest freshness even in my arid part of the world. Most areas of Texas have labored under a historic drought in recent years, so this little corner of my garden is the only place I consistently water and tend. While my xeric garden areas remind me of the resilience and strength of nature, this yoga deck oasis is my spot that reminds me of newness and vitality.

A MEDITATION FOR STRENGTH. If you are new to meditation and don't know where to begin, no worries – there are many types of "guided meditation" to be found, many of them with outdoor nature settings. One that I really like is the tree meditation (below), which can be helpful for anyone, but particularly those going through cancer treatment and struggling with health issues. You can do this meditation outside by a tree, or inside if the weather is not cooperating or you are more bedridden. I actually used a similar meditation during my first chemotherapy appointment to evoke feelings of strength and grounding. Please note: This is not worshipping a tree; this is simply using the imagery of a tree to feel strong, healthy and rooted.

1. *Sit outside with your back against a sturdy tree trunk, or if you are indoors, against a wall, imagining it to be a tree trunk behind you.*

2. *Close your eyes and take several deep breaths.*

3. *Imagine roots coming from the bottom of your legs or your spine, grounding and connecting you to the earth and your nourishment.*

4. *Now imagine branches extending from your head as well as your shoulders and arms, connecting you with the rest of the world and/or the Creator. Your branches give you air, light and energy.*

5. *As you continue to breathe deeply, imagine your breath coming from both sources, your roots and branches. Breathe air, energy and grounding into every cell of your body.*

6. *As you feel more and more grounded, relaxed and strong, feel free to make a request or visualize healing, comfort, strength or peace – whatever it is you need right now.*

7. *When you are ready, begin to pull your roots up from the earth and your branches back from the sky, breathing in deeply to become more aware of your surroundings. Give thanks for your strength and groundedness.*

8. *As you begin to open your eyes and stretch your limbs, be aware of any thoughts and feelings that come up for you, and write them down in a journal. As with dreams, it's easy to forget the experience the further away you get from it.*

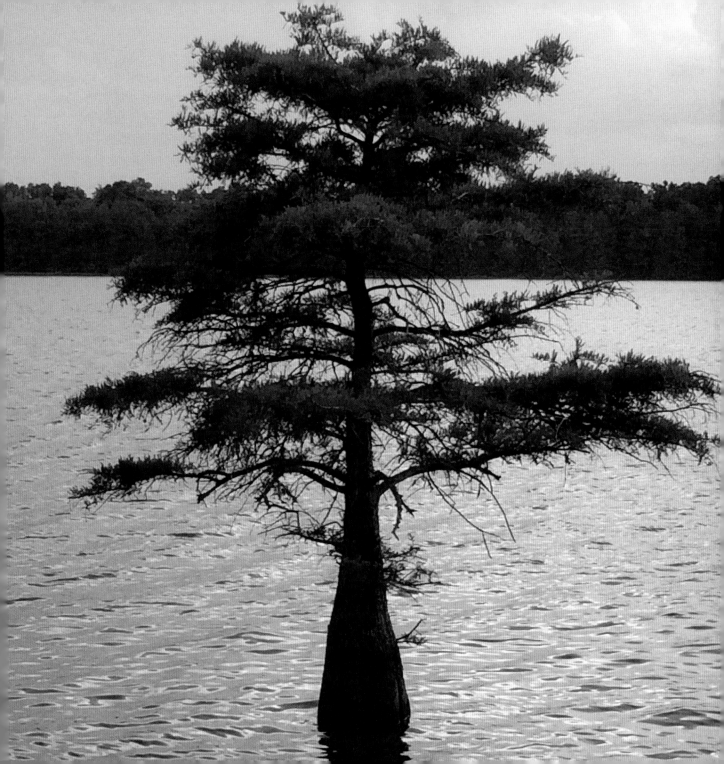

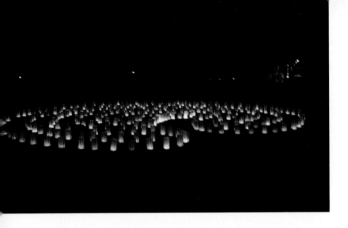

MY LABYRINTH. Another lovely way to pray or meditate is to walk a labyrinth. Labyrinths are different from mazes in that there is only one path to the center and back out again, whereas a maze is a left-brained puzzle of dead ends, twists and turns. Labyrinths have been a part of most mainstream religions for hundreds of years, and with their gentle paths swaying from one side of the labyrinth to another, they are conducive to creating a meditative mindset. I like to pray for others on the walk in to the center, stay silent when I pause at the center, and then humbly pray for my own needs on the walk out. One year, my fiancé and I lit hundreds of luminarias in our backyard and placed them along the pathway of a temporary labyrinth, then invited all our friends and family over for a contemplative evening.

Mantra

This word sounds very "Eastern" but is actually a fairly oft-used tool for meditation found in many mainstream spiritual practices. While much deeper explanations exist, the simplest one is that a mantra is a word or phrase that is repeated over and over again while a person is meditating. It can change each time — you can use mantras from your own religious or spiritual teaching, you can make up your own mantras, or you can listen closely to the hum or "mantra" of the world around you while meditating in your garden. When I was going through treatment and even now as I continue to recover, my mantra was, "My body is a place of strength, health and balance."

While you can certainly use mantras anywhere at any time, both aloud and silently in your head, practicing mantras outdoors, in the fresh air and with the sounds of your garden around you will have a much more profound effect. When we are outside, we are separated from more human-made distractions like phones, computers, appliances and housework, and we are reminded of the natural world that we were born into. There is a peace that surpasses our understanding and ability to articulate it.

Depending upon your spiritual or religious beliefs, there are mantras that will resonate with you. Here are a few examples of different mantras from various traditions:

- *Om, shanti, shanti, shanti* (Om, peace, peace, peace)
- *Lord Jesus, Son of God, have mercy on us.*
- *I ask for _____* (healing, love, strength, peace).
- *I am _____* (love, strong, a survivor, blessed).
- One word: *peace, love, hope, health, healing, courage,* repeated over and over (perhaps hold a meditative stone with the word etched into it in your hand while you meditate on the word).
- *Om* (this has no real translation, but can be interpreted as the sound of all the world or the voice of God).
- *Sabbe satta anigha hontu* (May all beings be free from physical suffering).
- *Hail Mary, full of grace.*

In creating your mantra and practicing it, there are a few guidelines to follow. These are not hard and fast rules, but rather guidelines to help the experience be as meaningful as possible.

1. Make it short and easy to remember.
2. Make it positive: rather than say, "I will not die from cancer," repeat "I will live with strength and courage," for example.
3. Set aside 20-30 minutes ideally for your mantra meditation, with a minimum of 15 minutes.
4. Make sure your environment is conducive to meditation – relatively quiet, warm and with low lighting. I've meditated outdoors in the winter, but made sure I was bundled up with

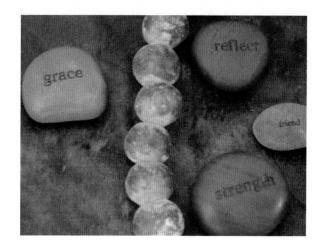

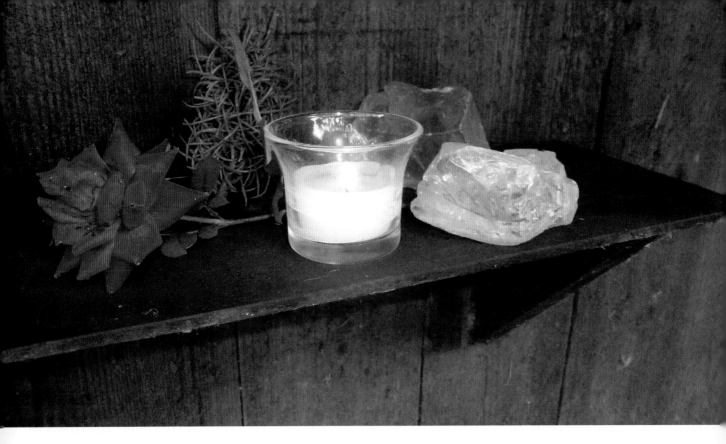

gloves on so I wouldn't get cold while my body was still. Remember to wear a warm hat, particularly if you have lost your hair to chemotherapy.

5. Sit or lie down in a comfortable position, one that you can hold for up to 30 minutes without too much shifting and rearranging. If you're outside, bring a pillow to sit on or a very comfortable chair to nestle into.

6. Close your eyes and breathe deeply for a few minutes to settle your body and mind before beginning your mantra.

7. When your mantra is complete, keep your eyes closed and your breathing deep for a few minutes as you are becoming more aware of your surroundings again.

Garden Altars

While admittedly this sounds a bit "churchy," think of the garden altar as a place to sit and give thanks, or to sit to meditate and pray, or to just sit. It's a physical place that you can create, a small but special area that you can go to when the need arises. It consists of two things: the physical "altar" and special items that you place on it. The altar itself can be the most humble of materials – an old tree stump, a fallen log, a garden bench, a large flat rock. It doesn't need to be elaborate; in fact, the more simple and organic it is, the better.

The items you bring to it should be special to you: candles for lighting, incense to burn, a small bowl of water to float a cut flower, rosary beads, meditation rocks with words carved into them, seashells from that vacation when you felt so relaxed, a small statuary from your tradition (The Virgin Mary, Buddha, etc.) – whatever speaks to you.

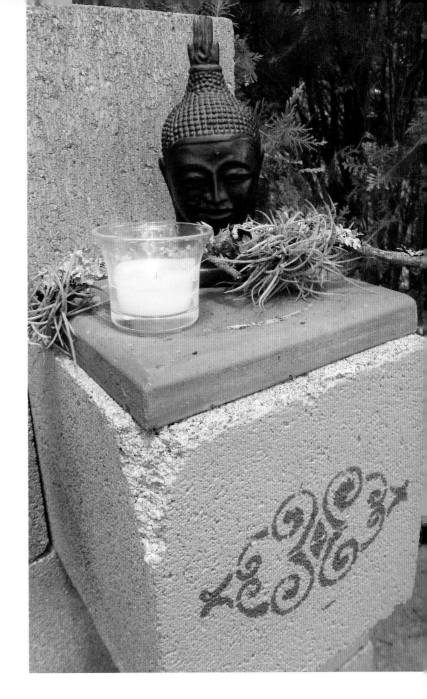

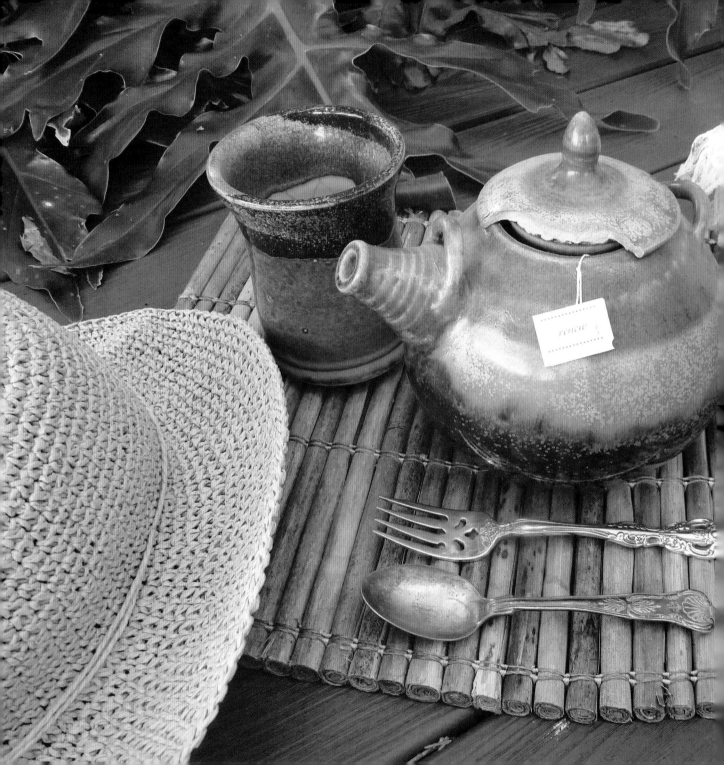

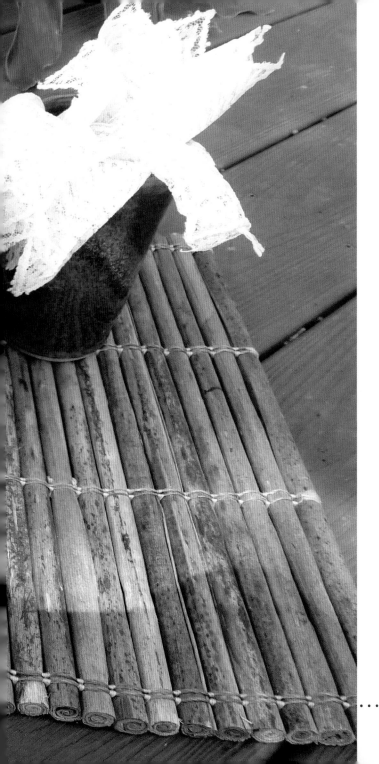

Change it out with the seasons, or start over every month with something new. Walk around your garden and pick up things that mean something to you and connect you to your garden.

I have a meditation altar inside my home, but it took this gardener getting diagnosed with breast cancer to create one outside. There is something so lovely and simple about a special place in my garden to sit and offer up a word of thanks or a request. In my tradition, time began in a garden, and I can think of no better place to reconnect and feel grounded and centered.

Wabi Sabi and the Tea Ceremony

Wabi: unpolished, imperfect, irregular beauty; the rustic elegance of things in their most austere, natural state.
Sabi: beauty that treasures the natural passage of time, and the patina that is created as a result; that which is true to the natural cycle of birth and death.

These Japanese words are closely related to the tea ceremony, and only in recent years have they come to be spoken as one singular phrase, *wabi sabi.* The tea ceremony has been loosely defined as "the art of everyday life," and is a way of achieving peace of mind through the simple preparation of tea in a quiet, serene (and possibly natural) environment. Everything in the tea ceremony has meaning, from the rustic tea bowl, the utensils, the aged kettle and the flower in the vase – all reminding us of the value of understated beauty and perfect imperfection.

I am no expert in Japanese culture or traditions, but this concept of *wabi sabi* speaks to me on many levels. As a gardener, I've experienced many moments of grace, strength and resilience in the garden when I see flowers springing up through concrete, poppy seeds blowing into my yard and blooming without aid, and the philodendron that came back after being covered in ice. The natural world is

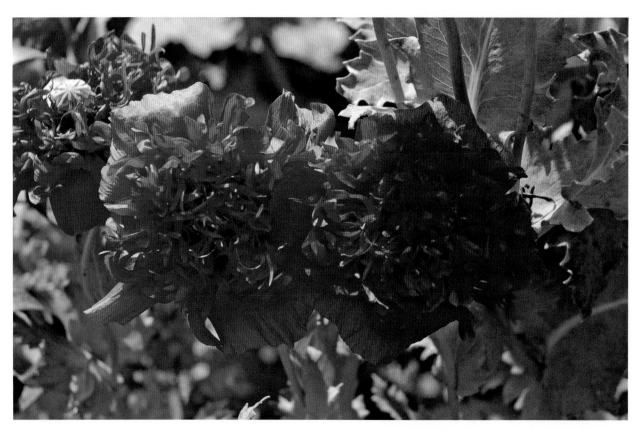

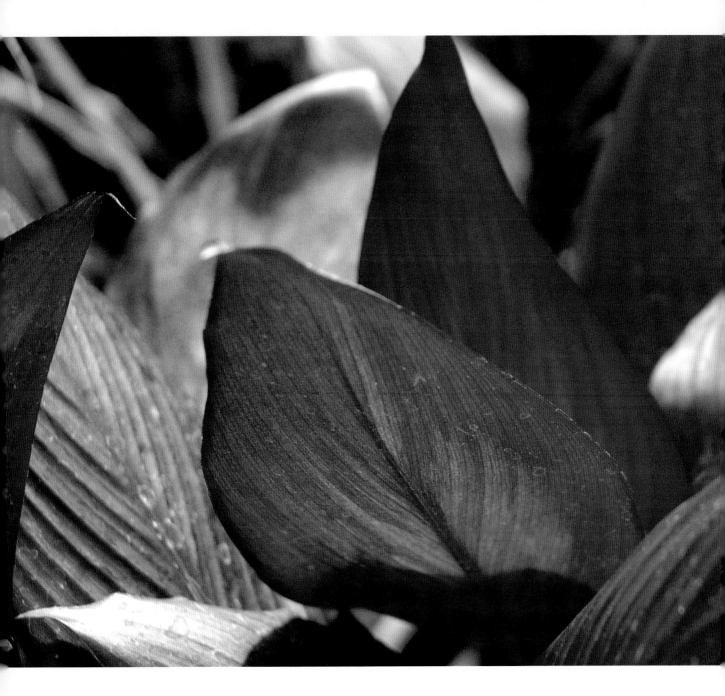

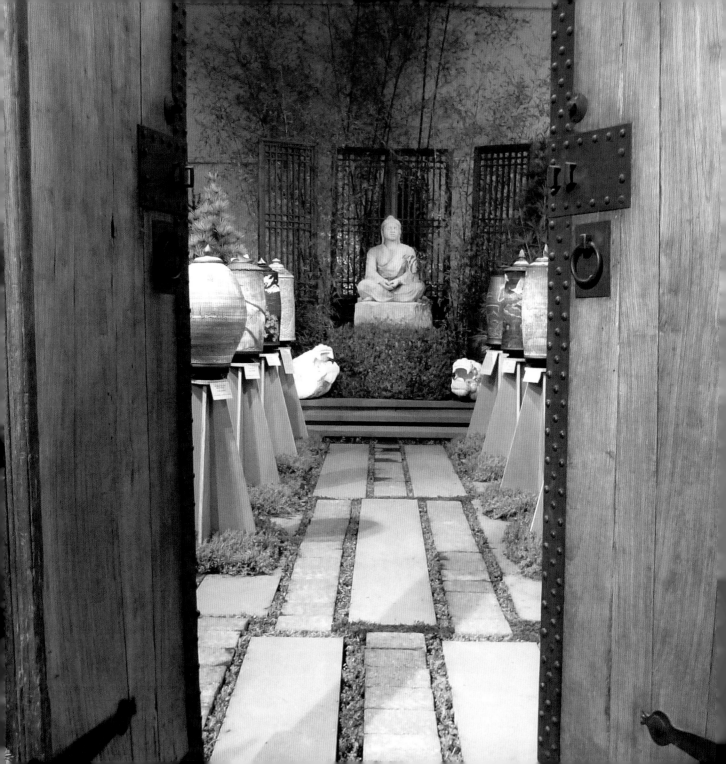

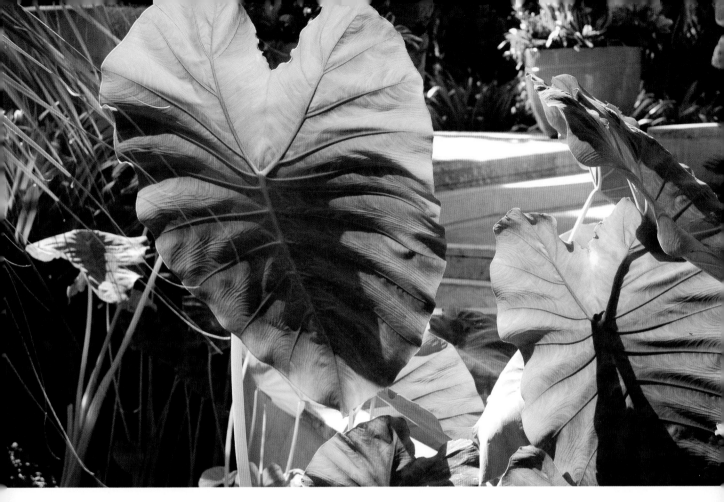

not always pretty, nor is it perfect (what if I didn't want those poppies in my yard?), but it reminds me of how every living thing seeks connection, balance and life. *Wabi sabi*, as expressed through the tea ceremony, is a simple and gracious way of honoring the imperfect while appreciating its beauty.

As you are going through your cancer treatment and recovery, think about embracing this concept by inviting a friend or two over for your own version of the tea ceremony, using your garden as the setting. You needn't be a cultural scholar to participate; I'm pretty sure our Japanese friends will appreciate

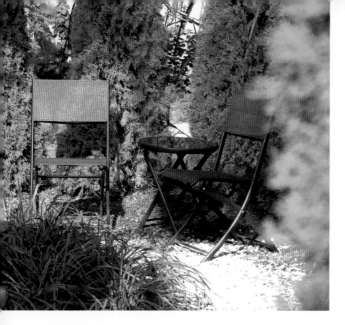

efforts to incorporate the meaning behind these elaborate ceremonies. The important thing, in my mind, is to make a distinction between a "tea party" and a "tea ceremony," as each has their place in our lives, relationships and gardens while honoring vastly different aspects of the world.

1. Invite your guest(s) for the ceremony in your garden. Explain to them what you are hoping to create (sense of peace, an honoring of your journey through treatment, acceptance that your life/body/health may not be perfect but it is nonetheless beautiful, connection with spirit, etc.). Help them understand that this is more of a quiet ritual than exuberant party.

2. Gather your utensils, taking care to choose them carefully. Perhaps you have a teapot that was your grandmother's, with a chip or two on its exterior. How about a couple of rustic pottery cups? And the copper teakettle with its aged patina, along with the bud vase that has scratches. These items, although imperfect, serve you with beauty and integrity while encouraging you to find respect and appreciation for where you are in your journey. Your scars, your hairless head, your imbalance, your radiation burns all speak to your strength and resilience.

3. Choose a spot in your garden that is peaceful and pretty – the middle of your vegetable garden, that space on your patio, the covered deck. Take your tea ingredients and utensils out to this place, where you've already placed your seating (simple lawn chairs and folding table, bistro set, cushions for the ground).

4. As you enjoy your tea together, use only words or actions/motions that are necessary – remember, everything in this ceremony, from the utensils to the location and your words, has meaning. Give thanks for the health you have, for the help you've received, for the peace you experience at that moment, for the friendships that have sustained you and for the garden that has brought you joy.

5. End the ceremony with whatever symbolic words or gestures from your tradition that make sense: Amen, prayer hands while saying *Namaste*, hands uplifted in gratitude, or a simple quiet hug.

*Ring the bells
that still can ring,
forget your perfect
offering.
There is a crack
in everything,
that's how the
light gets in.*
– Leonard Cohen

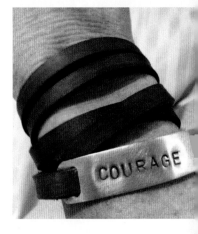

Wherever you are in your cancer journey, there is beauty around you. Whether you are a Stage 1 survivor or are in Stage 4 and living with ongoing treatment and uncertainties, the concepts of *wabi sabi* can help you to find peace, acceptance and gratitude. ∽

Survivor Spotlight

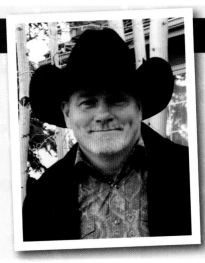

Name: Scooter

Diagnosed: 2013

Diagnosis: Throat Cancer

Stage: 4

Tip: Planting a seed in the soil, and watching it grow and bear fruit, is amazing. GOD Yahweh plants a seed in our hearts, in the same manner, to watch it grow and bear fruit. Praise and give Him glory for all that we have." *"Whatever you do, do your work heartily, as for the Lord rather than for men."* Col. 3:23

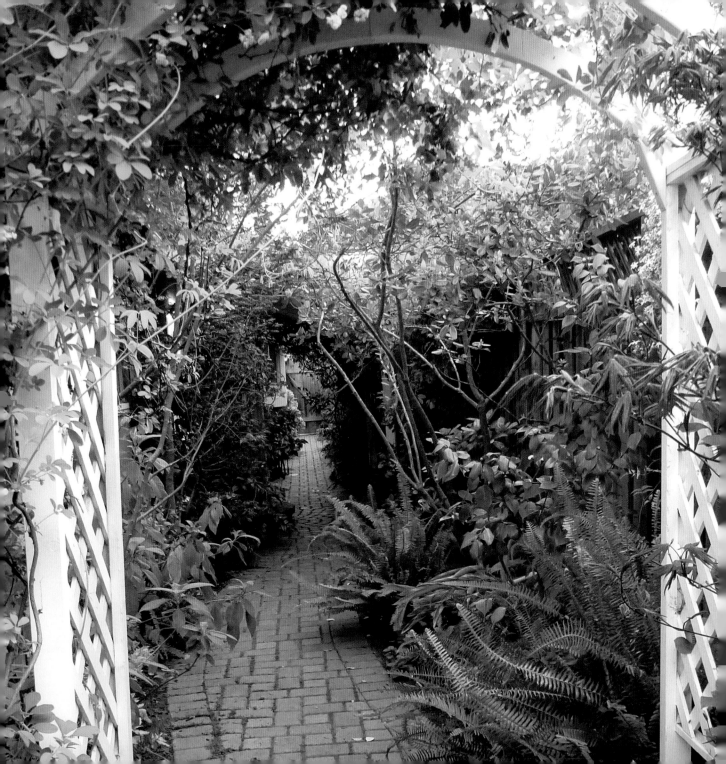

NINE

Renew Your Purpose

*B*efore your diagnosis, you may have had a pretty good idea of what you thought your life was about or what your purpose was. You thought you knew yourself pretty well, right? Surprise! It's Musical Chairs time, and you just missed the last chair. Down you go. Now, I'm the first to admit that a cancer diagnosis sucks – I won't even try to sugarcoat it. No amount of "Don't Worry; Be Happy" memes can change that. I believe in calling things for what they are, but I also believe that everything is an opportunity. For *what*, I'm not always sure, but it doesn't stop me from looking.

So let this opportunity sink in. Although it's a very difficult time, and for some, gravely life-threatening, it can also be a very deep, rich time in your understanding of yourself and of the world around you. Don't let this opportunity pass you by – let your garden remind you of who you are and what your purpose is. We might not even be talking about your overall life's purpose; perhaps it might be your purpose just for this one moment. But this one moment is what we have.

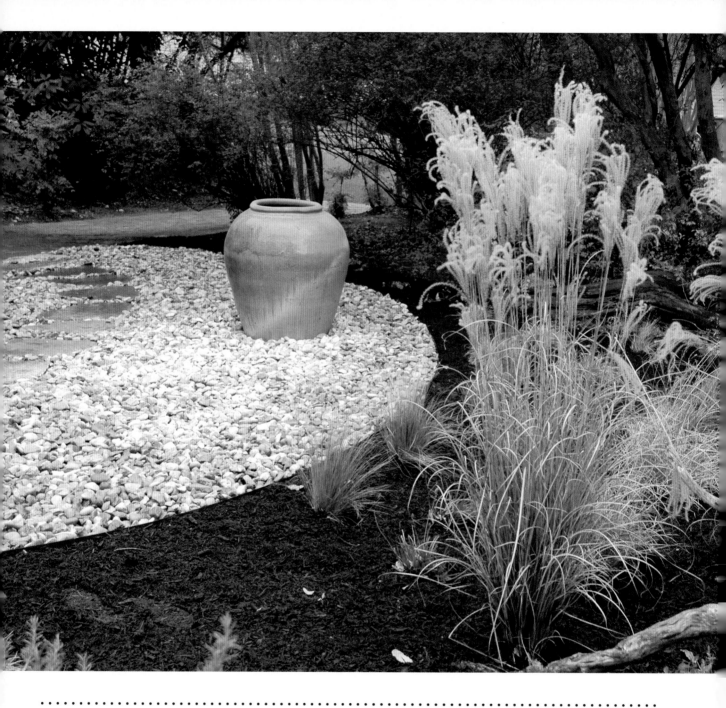

The Circle of Life

My father used to say corny things like, "Nobody's getting out of this life alive," and "Did you hear what's happening at the cemetery? Everyone's dying to get in." Groan. My father was a Lutheran pastor and retired Army chaplain, and he had a joke for everything. He also died of liver cancer in 1999 and was able to pull out his best puns up till the very end. Why do I tell you this? Because to live the most fully, you have to accept that life is a cycle and parts of it are finite. Whatever you believe about an "Afterlife," our world and the life within it is in a constant state of dying, rebirth and renewal. Just look at your garden if you doubt.

I don't say any of this to bum you out. If you've read this far in this book, you know that I like to encourage, and I'm a fairly optimistic person (some would say foolishly so). But from one cancer survivor to another, let's be real. If you want a book about simply having a "good attitude" during cancer treatment, you've probably bought the wrong book. (Or your best friend gave you the wrong book, in which case, you should probably find new people to hang out with that know you better.)

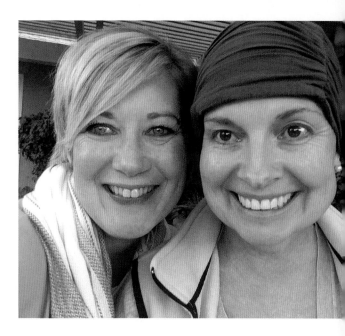

While I was writing this book, I took a trip to California to attend the San Francisco Flower and Garden Show. I stayed with my dear friend Rebecca, who is a landscape designer and writer, and who also happened to be going through her reconstruction after a double mastectomy. Anyone who knows Rebecca would describe her as funny, kind, bright-eyed and a positive person. Even her last name, Sweet, is cute. But while I was visiting her, she showed me a cancer book that someone had given her after her diagnosis. "Can you believe there are books like this out there?" she scoffed, "I'm tired of cute sayings and writings that make this sound like a walk in the park. You better write a different book!"

After we finished laughing, we had a great conversation about how difficult it is to strike that balance between taking all this seriously, but not *too* seriously. If all you are doing is making light of your cancer and cracking jokes, you can bet that it will come crashing down at some point, and it's not going to be pretty. But, on the other hand, if you are committed to doom and gloom, your quality of life will be fairly grim. So let's just be real.

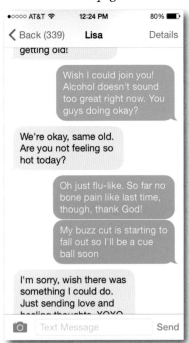

Part of being real is seeing that this circle of life, this finiteness, is not depressing. Again, look at your garden – last year's tomatoes didn't do so well, but this year's is looking to be a bumper crop. Those hostas may have

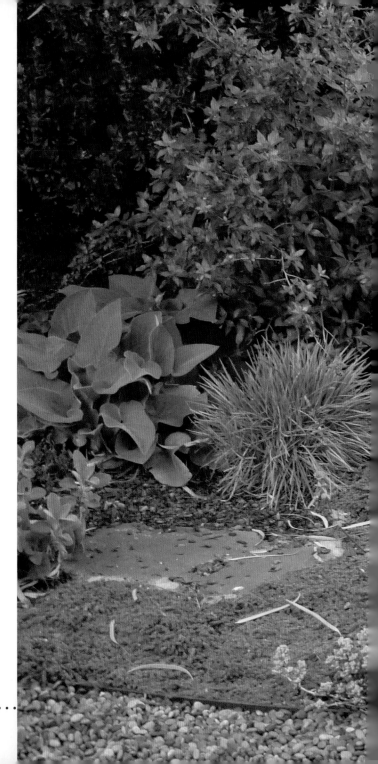

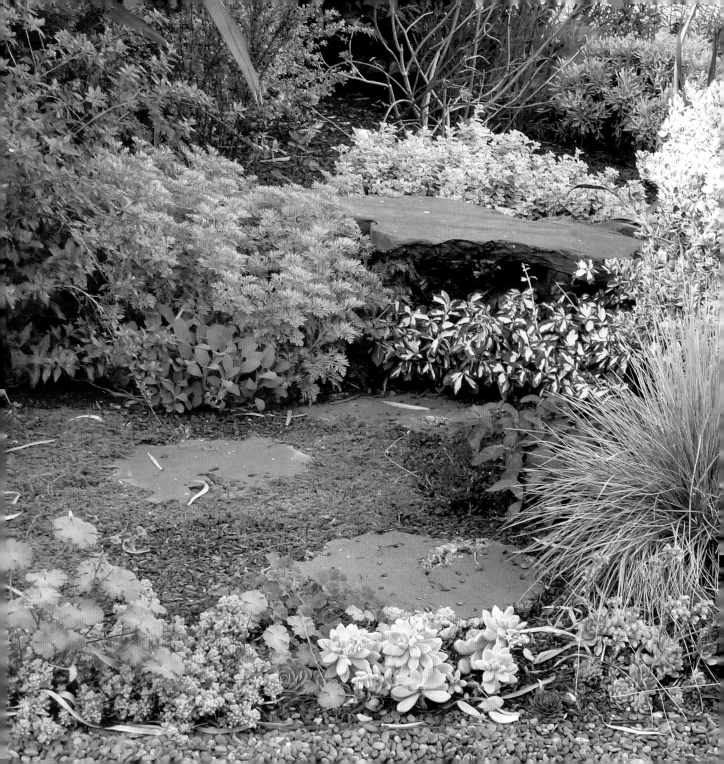

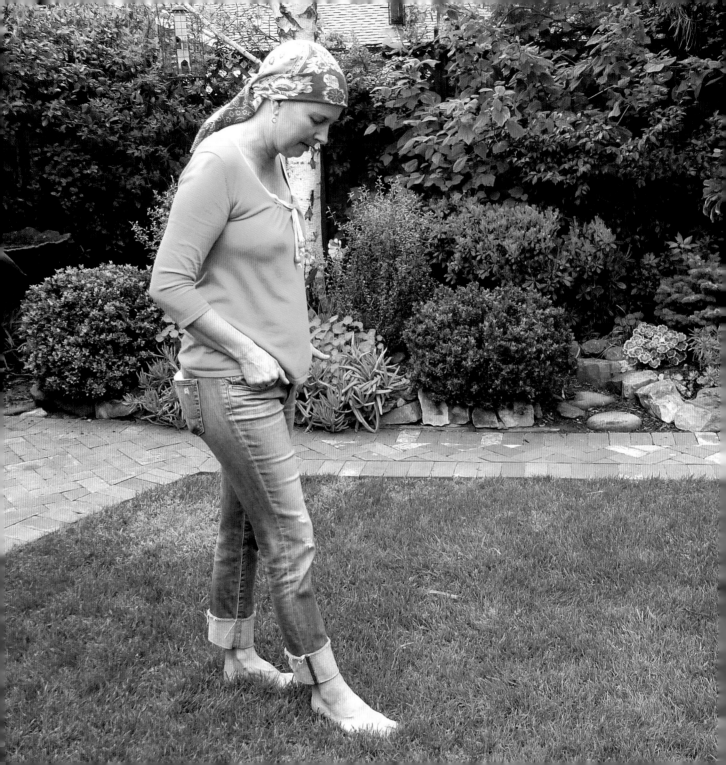

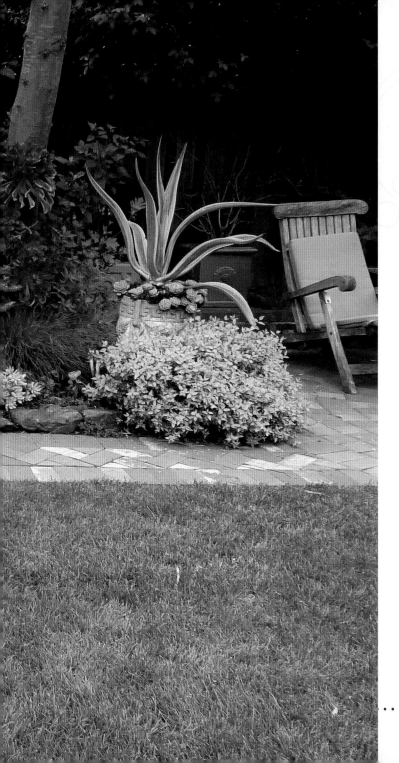

croaked because you gave them a little too much sun, but they'll be great in the compost pile. Years of drought in my area of Texas have suddenly been broken up by the most rain we've seen in recent memory (literally as I write this chapter). Life is a cycle. This encourages me, reassures me.

Some people reading this book are in remission. Some people are currently in treatment and are hoping for the best. Some of you might be in hospice care as a result of your treatment. We're all still survivors, because at this moment, we are, in fact, alive. With every breath you have, breathe it in with thanks and make it count.

Getting Grounded

After I finished treatment, I thought, "Wow, thank God I'm done with that. Let's get life back to normal now." Unwittingly, I was viewing my cancer treatment as a mere inconvenience, a short disruption in my life. It actually disrupted my Universe, and changed it forever. My expectation to begin living my life as though nothing had happened was rudely and swiftly challenged.

The first year after treatment consisted largely of what I had read it might – feeling tired, getting my hair back, dealing with foggy "chemo brain," rebuilding my strength. It was the second year, though, that threw me for a cosmic loop. My hormones finally crashed after being thrust into chemo-induced medical meno- pause, my brain seemed even foggier, my emotions were on a roller coaster ride from Hell and I saw no end in sight. This wasn't what I'd signed up for! The doctor who called me with my diagnosis said that I would feel better in a year. One year, not two and beyond.

It was during this time that I began working – with the blessing of my oncolo- gist – with a wonderful and gifted holistic practitioner, Dr. Robin Mayfield. Robin and I had been friends for several years, with both of us writing garden blogs and belonging to an Austin area garden blogging group. In fact, it's ironic that I'm mentioning Robin here, because her blog is about gardening in the Texas heat and harsh environment, and it's called "Getting Grounded: *It's not for sissies.*"

Cancer treatment and its recovery are, indeed, not for sissies. It kicked the snot out of me, and it continued to surprise

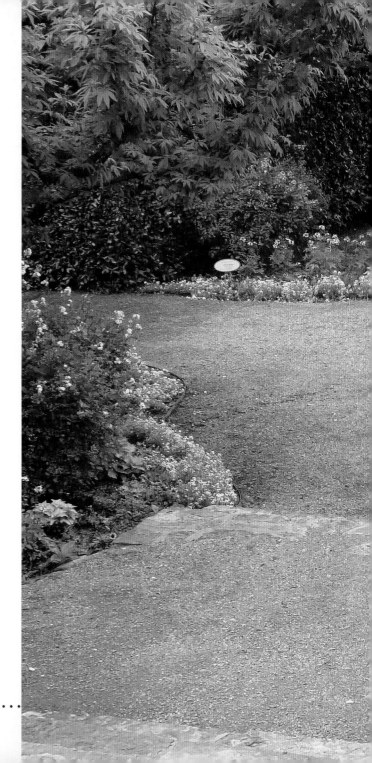

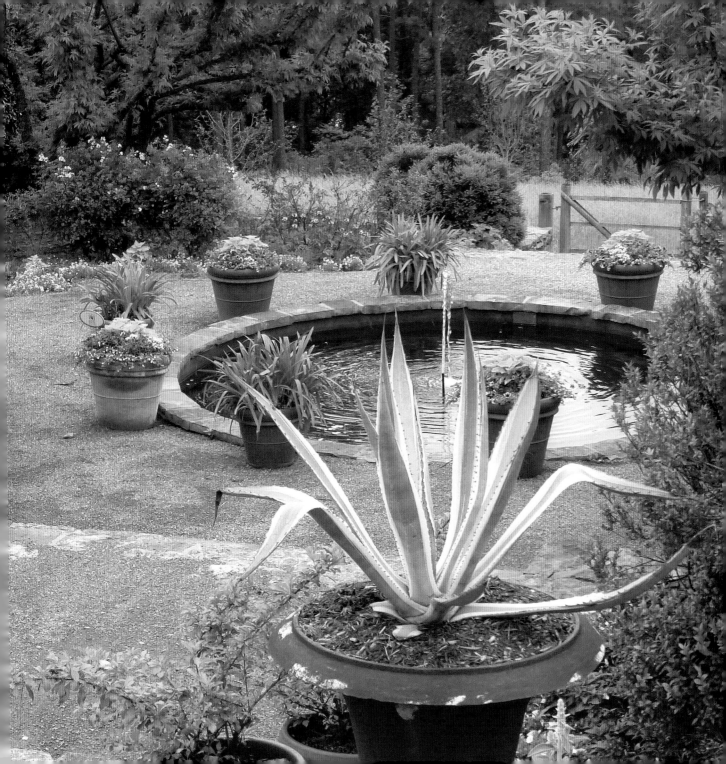

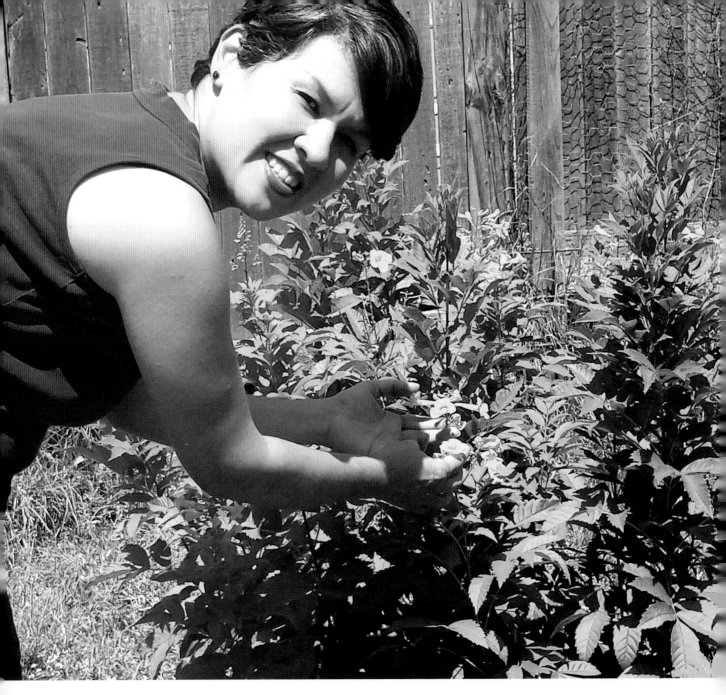

me that it took so long to recover. But Robin told me something that really resonated with me: every day, before you do anything else, get your cup of coffee or tea and go out into the garden. Don't do anything. Just check on your roses, appreciate the flowers you just planted, observe how many tomatoes are on the vine, greet your chickens. *Get grounded.* Feel the ground beneath your feet. It reminds you of who you are and where you came from.

For months, this was my ritual, and I treated it like my homework. Get grounded. This simple yet powerful ritual has a way of whispering in your ear, "Hey, just breathe. One day at a time. It's going to be okay."

But what, exactly, is getting "grounded" and how does it work? To answer that, think first about what it means to be "*un*grounded." That's where you're in a headspace of feeling angry, anxious, bitter, upset, distracted, unhappy. All those feelings are normal, but they also keep you from being in the here and now. They pull your mind away in a million different directions, and after a while you forget what it means to be *present*.

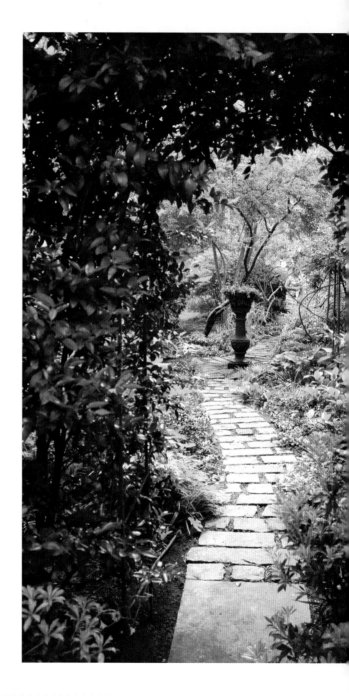

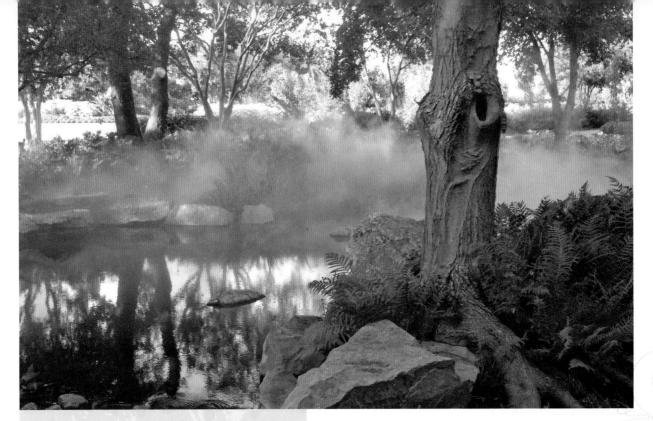

Ground Yourself

- Go outside.
- Get barefoot if possible.
- Walk on the soil or grass, not pavement.
- Feel the ground under your feet.
- Breathe in deeply.
- Be aware of your surroundings.
- Engage your senses (smell, touch, sight, hearing).

So get grounded. Get back to the basics. Take a few minutes for yourself, reminding yourself of what is real right now. Don't treat cancer and your treatment as merely an inconvenience, because you will be squandering away an opportunity to see a deeper meaning. Will you always feel like doing this? Of course not. But when you least feel like doing something is perhaps when it just may be the most beneficial to you.

Meaning and Essence

So...who *are* you, and where *did* you come from? One thing is for certain, you are not what you do. What you do is important, and it makes a difference, but it is not who you are. After my surgery, I ambled out into my garden, somewhat shocked at how difficult my surgery had been. I walked around, aimless, feeling stripped of everything. I was not a writer (or so I thought), I was not a designer, I was not a landscaper. All of these labels sounded so hollow and meaningless at the time.

But somehow, the thought "I am a gardener" rang true. A *gardener* – the simplest and most humble interpretation of most of my professional and personal life. Also the most profound. A *gardener* – I tend, I care, I nurture. I am a part of Creation.

In my religious tradition, a garden is where earthly life began. Every morning of my recovery – and we are always in recovery to some degree, aren't we? – I took joy in remembering that. If time and life as we know it began in a garden, then this was the best place for me. It was enough; more than enough. Something more ancient than I could ever really conceive of was surrounding me with its beauty, its wisdom, its experience. It felt safe.

Your garden will remind you of who you are, and to Whom you belong, however it is that you express that.

Trust

Yeah, this is a tough one. After a cancer diagnosis, you trust that the diagnosis is correct. You trust that the surgeon removed all of your cancer, that chemotherapy will zap every cancer cell in your body and that radiation will finish off any stragglers that dare to still hover. You trust that the medication you are taking is going to help your 5-year survival rate.

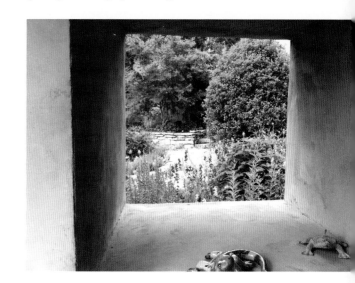

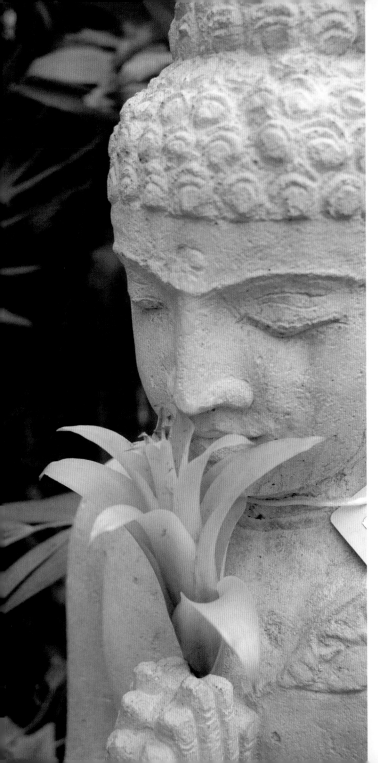

For me, the whole experience far surpassed merely *trust*. It was a leap of faith. Actually, it was a nosedive off a cliff, really hoping my chute would open, and if it didn't, that there would be somebody down there who would catch me. Talk about white-knuckling. Sky-diving has never been on my Bucket List, and for a very good reason.

But something I've observed over the years in my garden is that nature works to "right" things, doesn't it? There are checks and balances for all sorts of things that can go wrong. For example: Too many aphids? Ladybugs to the rescue! Not enough nitrogen in the soil? Let legumes add it back in. While the theory that nature is inherently always in balance has been generally discredited, there is plenty of evidence to suggest that Mother Nature often knows best, and has many systems in place to correct problems, errors and deficiencies.

The takeaway here, for me, is to trust the process. Western minds tend to be very solution-oriented, to the point that we often forget to be aware of the process it takes to get to the solution. Yes, I'd have loved to have fast-forwarded through chemotherapy, and to have skipped lymphedema altogether, but that wasn't my reality. Was I going to hate every day that I was in treatment, refuse to see any beauty around me, or never laugh again? Was I going to curl up and stop living?

Now lest you think that I'm simply saying "Have a positive attitude," let me tell you that I am not a big proponent of that theory. Positive attitudes are fine, I guess, but there is a limit to what one can be positive about. Someone told me once during treatment, "If you have a positive attitude, you'll get through it just fine." I am pretty sure I grumbled back, "Yeah, I'm pretty positive it's going to suck to lose my hair."

Positive attitudes don't take bad things into account, they simply encourage you to whistle past the graveyard and only see the good things. Our gardens don't teach us that, do they? They teach us to *acknowledge* the difficulties, the traumas, to seek the balance, to fix what we can and then let the stuff we can't fix *go*.

Our gardens are huge proponents of living in reality, and with what is. So, let this time in your life make a difference. What kind of a difference is totally up to you. ∼

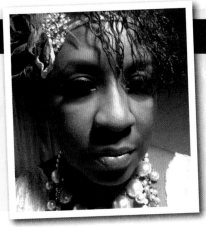

Survivor Spotlight

Name: Donna Renae
Age at diagnosis: 36 and 43
Diagnosis: Breast Cancer and Ovarian Cancer
Tip: Don't feel guilty for taking time out for yourself. I made a small meditation seating spot on my front porch. All you need is cute folding chairs, a folding table with an inspirational book or display, and a plant.

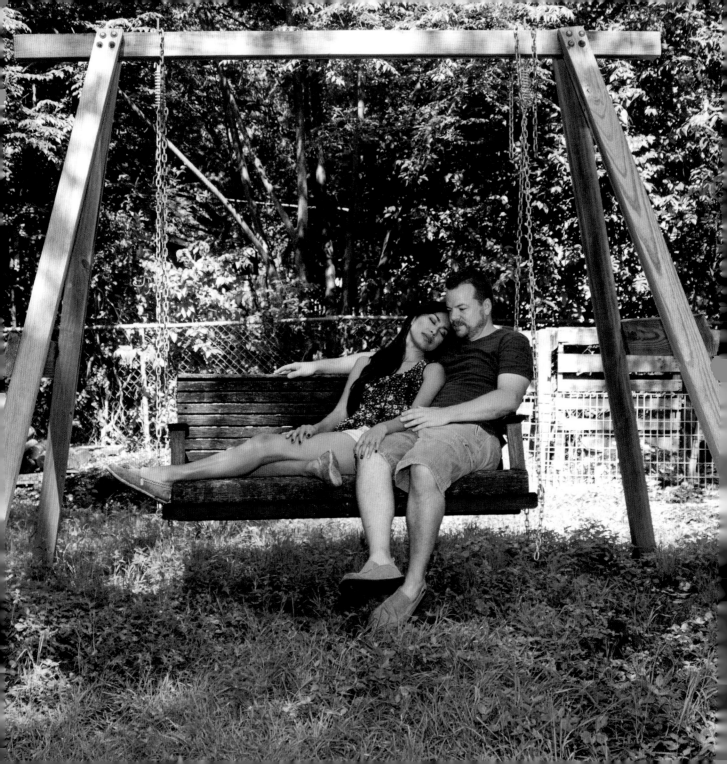

TEN

Be Present in Time

*O*ur human minds always want to second-guess the past and predict the future, and even more so after a cancer diagnosis, right? "Why didn't I go in for a check-up earlier? Why did I skip that mammogram/colonoscopy/annual checkup? I knew I wasn't feeling right. Will I die? Will my children be okay? Who will remember me?"

These are difficult thoughts to have, and I remember having a surreal feeling as I realized I was having them. This surely couldn't be happening to *me*. Yet, it was. And each time I allowed my thoughts to go down one of those rabbit holes, I felt more and more hopeless, panicked and despondent.

As heartbreaking – and as normal – as these thoughts are, and as difficult as it is to keep your mind from going there, it's much healthier to remain in the here and now, to be present in time – *this* time. Right now, I am alive. Right now, I have my family with me. Right now, I have a great medical team. Right now, I *am*.

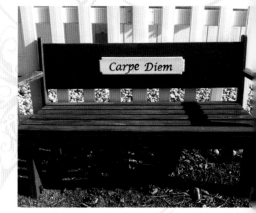
Carpe Diem

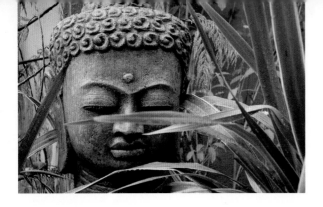

Get Zen

I was watching "The Karate Kid" recently and discovered a new appreciation for the "wax on, wax off" ritual that drove Daniel, The Kid, nuts.

Miyagi: First, wash all car. Then wax. Wax on...

Daniel: Hey, why do I have to...?

Miyagi: Ah ah! Remember deal! No questions!

Daniel: Yeah, but...

Miyagi: Hai!

[makes circular gestures with each hand]

Miyagi: Wax on, right hand. Wax off, left hand. Wax on, wax off. Breathe in through nose, out the mouth. Wax on, wax off. Don't forget to breathe, very important.

[walks away, still making circular motions with hands]

Miyagi: Wax on, wax off. Wax on, wax off.

What was the point of this? That rote tasks can become the tool through which many other teachings and truths are revealed or realized. Daniel doesn't see this at first, and when he expresses his frustration, Miyagi reveals that Daniel has been learning defensive karate blocks through muscle memory learned by performing the chores.

I know what you're thinking right now. "I'm going through cancer treatment; I don't have the time or energy to learn 'truths' and 'teachings.' Seriously, Jenny?" Yep, super serious. When something develops in your body that could potentially kill you, don't you think that's the *best* time to learn truths and teachings? Look, even if none of us developed cancer, we still don't know how much time we have left on this earth, so get about learning the truths and teachings, my friend.

About a year after I finished treatment, I was so hungry one day that I was scarfing down a sandwich. My friend Todd joked, "Dude, slow down. You're going to choke and kill yourself." I said, "Wouldn't that be ironic? I get through cancer treatment and then die because I was stupid and choked on a sandwich? If that happens, you have my permission – no, you are *obligated* – to make fun of me at the funeral. In fact, serve sandwiches and have a sandwich-eating contest."

I joke, but I am also serious. I could actually get through cancer treatment and die the next day of something totally unrelated. You could, too. Anyone could. It's the way things work sometimes. So, learn the dang truths and teachings.

I love how our gardens teach us the truths and teachings through rote chores. During your treatment and healing, go out into your garden and do some rote, zenlike chores. Whatever it is for you that doesn't require much thought, that's what you do. You can do it in your sleep. Keep doing it. Notice the images, thoughts or connections that come up for you during

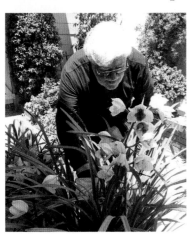

this time, and don't judge them. Don't even linger on them; just notice them and keep doing what you're doing.

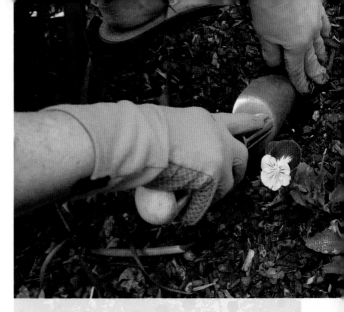

Rote Garden Chores

- Watering
- Hand weeding
- Hoeing
- Turning the compost
- Walking a labyrinth
- Deadheading flowers

This makes the second time in this book that I've mentioned labyrinths, and I want to make sure I define what it is and why I think they are so valuable. Labyrinths are often confused with mazes, but they are very different. While mazes are left-brained puzzles containing dead ends and false turns, labyrinths are a right-brained activity that requires no decision-making. Labyrinths have one pathway to the center, with the exact same pathway leading back out again. Mazes are fun; labyrinths are enriching. There's an old saying, "You can't get lost in a labyrinth, but you might just find yourself."

Metaphorically, labyrinths reflect the path of illness and recovery – that, despite the many uncertainties of our illness, if we are diligent and stay the course, we will arrive at our goal. But there has also been research into the back-and-forth bilateral motion of the walking that suggests that brain activity is calmed when bodies participate in it. Think about pacing, reading, knitting, all those things that require a back-and-forth motion and that also calm us.

If you're intrigued about labyrinths, do a quick Google search to locate one in your area, as churches and hospitals often have them at their facilities. If you want to make one in your own garden, here is a quick demonstration on how the pathways are laid out.

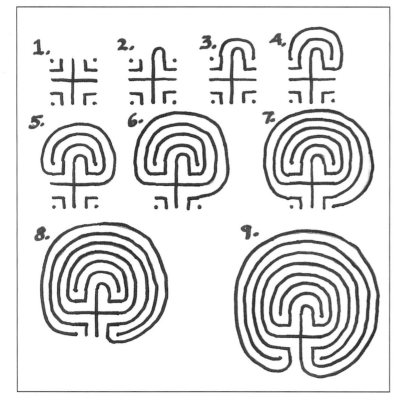

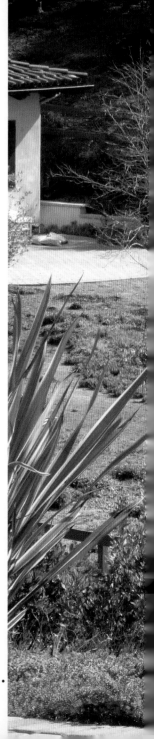

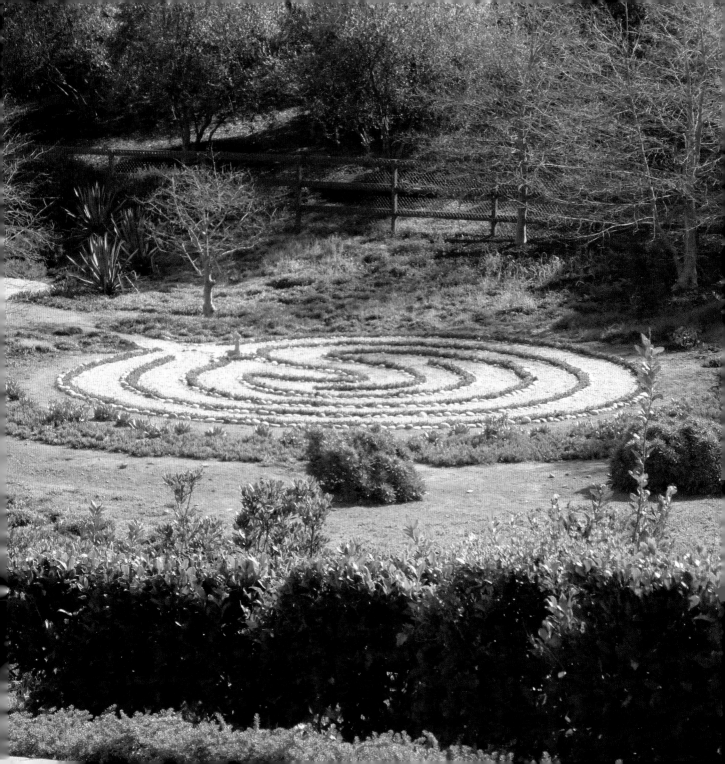

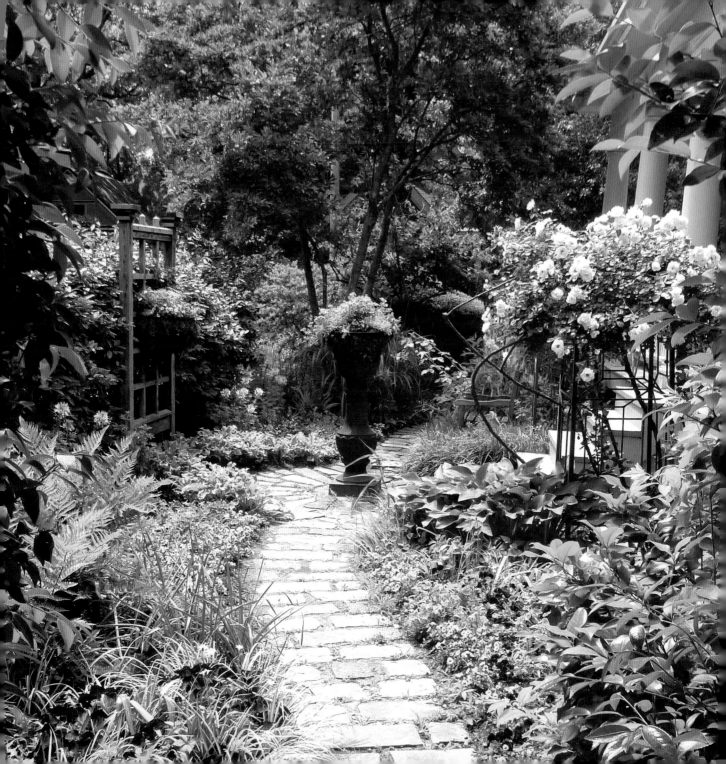

Acceptance

There's a saying I read recently, "Flowers don't compare themselves to the flowers next to them. They just bloom." Easier said than done, of course, but flowers teach us acceptance of ourselves, our situation, our bodies, our neighbors and our world. They are not attached to an outcome; they spend zero time thinking, "Hmm...wonder if that butterfly will come over to me."

My fiancé, Brett, has spent some time studying Buddhist teachings, and it took me a very long time to begin to understand one of them. He would talk about the importance of being "unattached," as in "not being attached to an outcome or a thing." For a long time, that sounded lifeless and cold to me – why is it bad to be attached to something or someone? I'm certainly attached to my boys, Max and Luke, for example.

But this teaching means that your ability to be okay, to function and to live, is not dependent upon a particular thing happening. It doesn't mean that you don't care, that things or people aren't important to you or that you don't try to affect a positive change. It simply means that

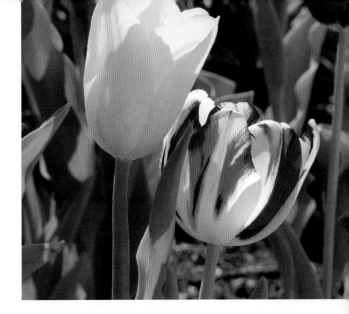

you understand that the change you are looking for may not actually happen. This teaching became a very profound one to me while I was in treatment, as you can obviously relate.

I accept that cancer has been a part of my life. I accept that I have done what I can do in order for it to not come back into my life in a more permanent way (surgery, chemotherapy, radiation, medication). I accept that my life is different now. And I accept that cancer may come back. I can't live in a headspace that says, "What if..."

So, acceptance and detachment. Take a cue from your garden. Be the flower.

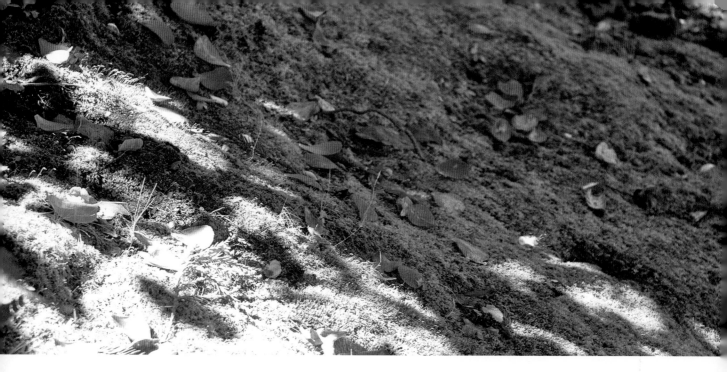

Allow

There are plenty of times when you'll need to do things, or accomplish things, in your garden, but today may not be that time. Today, let your garden be a place where you can just...be.

My father, Richard, was diagnosed with liver cancer in early 1999. He'd been exposed to Agent Orange during the Vietnam War where he was a chaplain in the Army, and years later, he developed cirrhosis of the liver. He didn't respond to treatment very well, and soon enough was dealing with liver cancer. So we moved him from his house in San Antonio, Texas, to my house in New Braunfels, Texas, to live out the rest of his days. Turns out, those days were numbered.

But there was one thing that stood out in my mind about one of those numbered days that I often remember with a bitter-sweet feeling. Dad was losing a major function pretty much every day at that point, and on one of the last days that he was able to walk unaided, rain started to fall outside. Dad ambled out onto my deck with his hands outstretched, letting the rain fall on his face.

One of my sisters began to get upset, and attempted to usher Dad back inside. "Let him be," I said, "This will be the last time he feels rain on his face." And, amazingly, it wasn't sad to watch this. I not only felt honored to be caring for my father in his last days, I was gladdened that I could witness such a scene. My father was an avid gardener, and I can only imagine what that gentle rain felt like on his face. Rather than cloister himself inside to live out his days in misery, he embraced what was happening in that moment. I have never witnessed someone *really living* in the moment as I did that day.

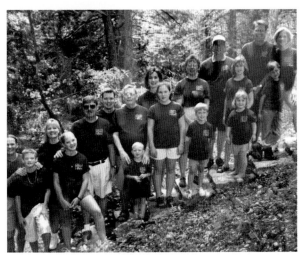

My father, surrounded by his family at our family reunion, a month before he died.

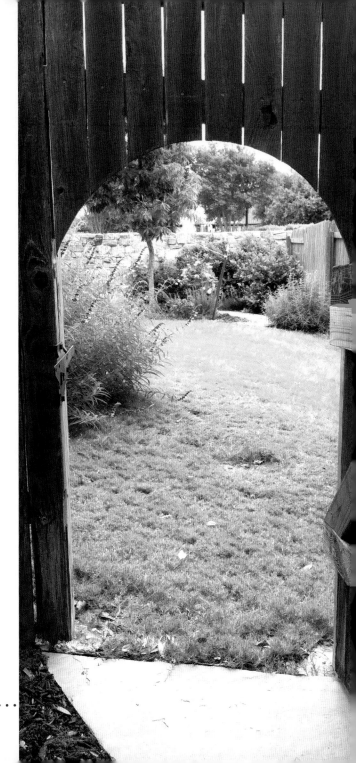

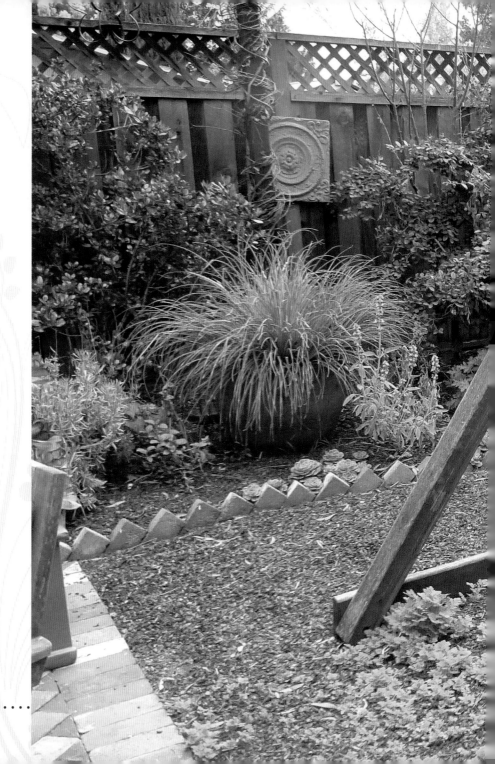

I've had moments of that myself, and it's almost always when I'm outside. Nature is a beautiful host to simply "allowing" whatever is, to be. I'm often amazed at how difficult that is to do, but I find it much easier in my garden. Sometimes I take my coffee or cocktail out to the garden and just sit or recline on the chaise lounge, breathing in the air and listening to the garden's sounds.

Getting out in the garden to simply "be" can be a solo trip or one with a loved one. Swing on your kids' swingset, snuggle up with your beloved (who's gone through a lot during your treatment, too), or if there's a light activity like reading that is relaxing to you, go ahead and do that. I've also found that hanging out in the garden with my pets is healing – dogs in particular are so good at just "being."

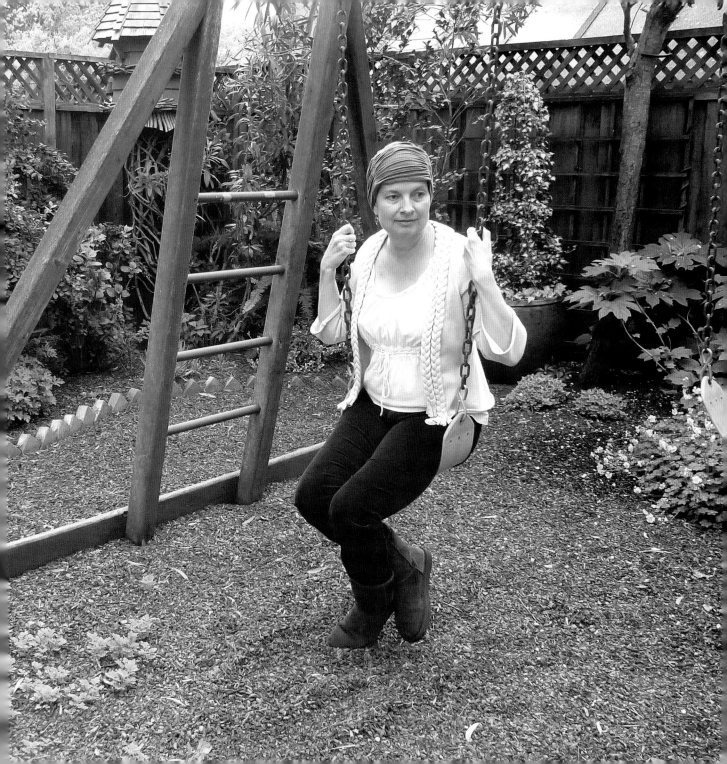

Animals

Most of my friends have pets, and these furry companions are the best at just hanging out and living in the moment.

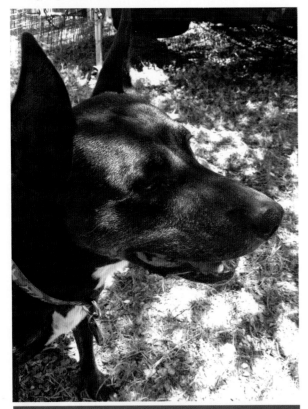

Live in the moment. Live with gusto. It's okay if you get bloodied or scarred, if it's for a good reason. Be loyal. Love the life you have. Have fun with your friends. Take naps. Learn to receive. Drink water. Shake it off. Get dirty. Be yourself. Stretch a lot. Love unconditionally. Go for walks. Trust your instincts. Get lots of rest.

We adopted our dog Pip when I was going through treatment, and it was the greatest gift for all of us. Pip had survived two high-kill shelters in California before somehow making her way to a wonderful rescue group outside of Austin. She was 5 at the time, and a perfect mix of protective guard dog and companion. She was not at all a clingy dog – in fact, we often called her a "Redneck Cowgirl" because of her fierce independence.

Yet, Pip would follow me around on the days when I was feeling my worst during treatment. She'd lie at my feet, sit patiently outside the bathroom door when I was sick, and stick to my side when I began having awful side effects from my medications. Sadly, we had to put her down while I was writing this book – she was diagnosed with lymphoma and went downhill within days, but the lessons I learned from that dog are profound and priceless.

So here's to all of our animal friends who see us through our tears, our treatments, our illnesses and our fears. I thank them for teaching us to really live, to be happy and peaceful in spite of our circumstances, and to have the courage to take risks in the midst of uncertainty.

seize the moment!

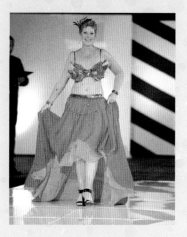

After I finished treatment, I modeled a bra to raise funds for the Breast Cancer Resource Center of Austin, and I modeled again the following year. It's not easy to get up on a 30-foot-long runway in front of hundreds of people, with flashing cameras and in a bra, but you gotta seize the moment sometimes.

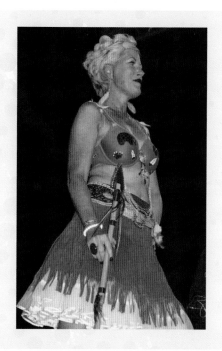

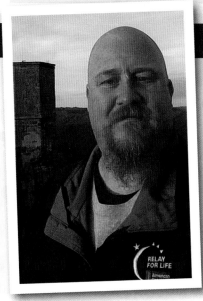

Survivor Spotlight

Name: Chris

Age at diagnosis: 37

Diagnosis: Testicular Cancer (Embryonal Carcinoma / Mature Teratoma)

Stage: IIIB (T1N0M1aS2)

Tip: I did a lot of walking in silence when I was going through treatment. Just being outside and moving was important for me. I saw and felt things differently than I ever had before. Every little breeze or flower filled me with hope and determination to continue. Getting out for a walk each day - however short - helped restore me.

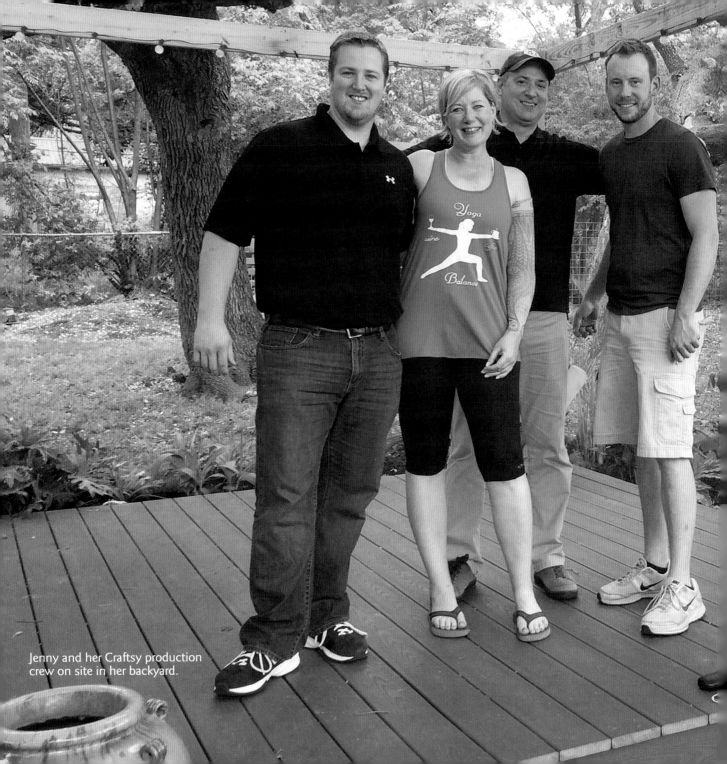

Jenny and her Craftsy production crew on site in her backyard.

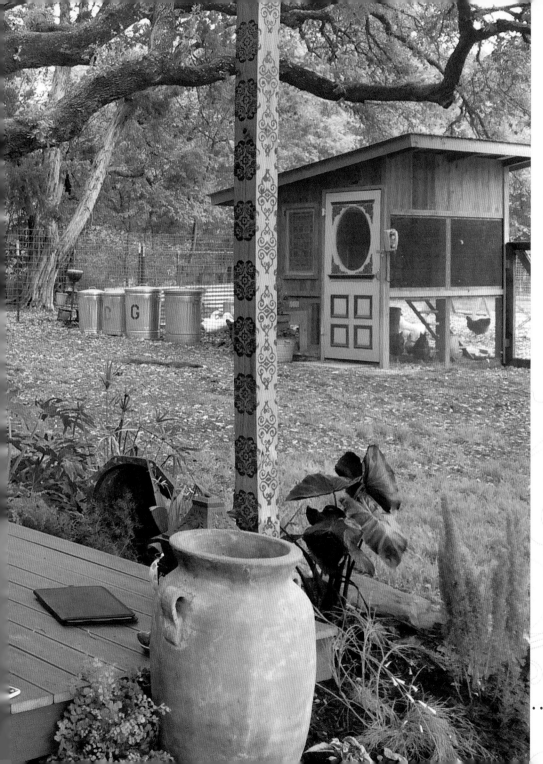

While writing this book, I had a health scare that resulted in my getting a chest scan to rule out metastatic breast cancer. Everything turned out well with a clean scan, but during that time I was to begin filming an online garden design class with Craftsy.com. I decided that no matter what the scan revealed, I would continue with filming the Craftsy class, not because I'm Wonder Woman, but because I want to take advantage of the opportunities life presents to me. I want to really live.

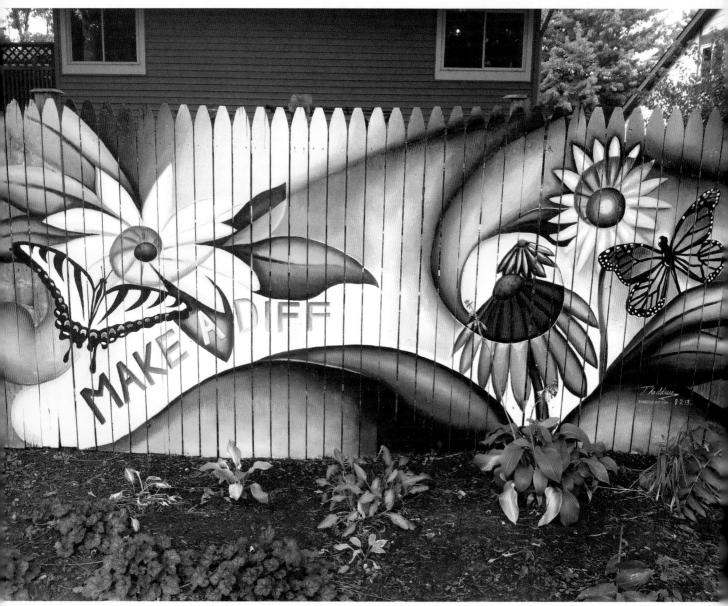

My friend Shawna's personal and professional motto is "Make a Dif!"
Make a difference for yourself every day and, over time, it adds up.

RESOURCES

BOOKS

(nonfiction)

100 Perks of Having Cancer: Plus, 100 Tips for Surviving It! by Florence Strang and Susan Gonzalez. Basic Health Publications, Inc., 2013.

Dr. Susan Love's Breast Book, by Dr. Susan Love, et al. De Capo Lifelong Books, 2015.

The Emperor of All Maladies: A Biography of Cancer, by Siddhartha Mukherjee. Scribner, 2011.

American Cancer Society Complete Guide to Nutrition for Cancer Survivors, Second Edition: Eating Well, Staying Well During and After Cancer, edited by Barbara L. Grant, Abby S. Bloch, Kathryn K. Hamilton and Cynthia A. Thomson. American Cancer Society, 2010.

There's No Place Like Hope: A Guide to Beating Cancer in Mind-Sized Bites, by Vickie Girard. Compendium Publishing & Communications, 2008.

The Herb Lover's Spa Book, by Sue Goetz. St. Lynn's Press, 2015.

Heaven is a Garden, by Jan Johnsen. St. Lynn's Press, 2014.

(fiction)

The Fault in Our Stars, by John Green. Penguin Young Readers Group, 2014.

All the Light We Cannot See, by Anthony Doerr. Scribner, 2014.

WEBSITES

American Cancer Society – cancer.org

American Lung Association – lung.org

Association of Online Cancer Resources – acor.org

Breast Cancer Resource Centers – (There is no central organization, but some regions have local breast cancer resource centers; best to search online to find one nearby.)

Caring Bridge – caringbridge.org

Leukemia & Lymphoma Society – lls.org

The Livestrong Foundation – livestrong.com

Mayo Clinic – mayoclinic.org

MD Anderson – mdanderson.org

National Institutes of Health – nih.gov

National Cervical Cancer Coalition – nccc-online.org

Ovarian Cancer Institute – ovariancancerinstitute.org

Prostate Cancer Foundation – pcf.org

The Skin Cancer Foundation – skincancer.org

Stupid Cancer – stupidcancer.org

Susan G. Komen – komen.org

RESOURCES

GARDEN TOOLS

Ames Tools
1380 Beverage Drive, Suite W
Stone Mountain, GA 30083
(800) 303-1827
amestools.com

Bahco
www.bahco.com – to find the nearest dealer
that carries bahco tools

Corona Tools
22440 Temescal Canyon Rd
Corona, CA 92883
(800) 847-7863
coronatoolsusa.com

Fiskars
2537 Daniels St.
Madison, WI 53718 USA
(866) 348-5661
fiskars.com

Flexzilla
Legacy Manufacturing Company
6281 North Gateway Drive
Marion, IA 52302
(800) 645-8258
flexzilla.com

Green Heron Tools
P.O. Box 71
New Tripoli, PA 18066
(610) 844-5232
greenherontools.com

Radius Garden Tools
P.O. Box 2506
Ann Arbor, MI 48106
(734) 222-8044
radiusgarden.com

GARDEN HATS, GLOVES, CLOTHING & SHOES

Bogs Footwear
(877) 321-BOGS (2647)
bogsfootwear.com

BugsAway Clothing
ExOfficio, Inc.
4202 6th Ave South
Seattle, WA 98108
(800) 644-7303
exofficio.com

Coolibar
(800) 926-6509
coolibar.com

Foxgloves, Inc.
1250 North Avenue
Beacon, NY 12508
To order: (888) 322-4450
Other: (845) 831-7300
foxglovesinc.com

RESOURCES

Gardener's Supply Company
128 Intervale Road
Burlington, VT 05401
(800) 876-5520
gardeners.com

Garden Girl
(866) 610-5459
gardengirlusa.com

Peaceful Valley
PO Box 2209
125 Clydesdale Court
Grass Valley, CA 95945
(888) 784-1722
groworganic.com

Tilley Endurables
3176 Abbott Road, Building A
Orchard Park, New York 14127
(800) 363-8737
tilley.com

Tula Hats
(888) 232-4287
tulahats.com

Wonder Grip
3070 Bristol Street, Ste 440
Costa Mesa, CA 92626
wondergrip.net
(949) 326-8583

COMPRESSION SLEEVES

Jobst
BSN medical Inc.
5825 Carnegie Blvd.
Charlotte, NC 28209
(800) 537-1063
jobst-usa.com

Juzo
juzousa.com – to find the nearest dealer that carries Juzo products

LympheDIVAs
7 North Street, Suite 205
Pittsfield, MA 01201
(866) 411-DIVA (3482)
lymphedivas.com

PLANT & BULB CATALOGUES

Annie's Annuals & Perennials
740 Market Ave.
Richmond, CA 94801
(510) 215-3301
anniesannuals.com

Bluestone Perennials
7211 Middle Ridge Road
Madison, OH 44057
(800) 852-5243
bluestoneperennials.com

RESOURCES

Bonnie Plants
1727 Hwy 223
Union Springs, Alabama 36089
bonnieplants.com

Brent & Becky's Bulbs
7900 Daffodil Lane
Gloucester, VA 23061
(804) 693-3966
brentandbeckysbulbs.com

W. Atlee Burpee Co.
300 Park Ave, Warminster, PA 18974
(215) 674-4900
burpee.com

Gurney's Seed & Nursery Co.
P.O. Box 4178
Greendale, IN 47025-4178
(812) 260-2153
gurneys.com

High Country Gardens
223 Ave D, Suite 30
Williston, VT 05495
(800) 925-9387
highcountrygardens.com

Michigan Bulb Co.
P.O. Box 4180
Lawrenceburg, IN 47025-4180
(812) 260-2148
michiganbulb.com

Proven Winners
111 E Elm St, Ste D
Sycamore, IL 60178
(815) 895-8130
provenwinners.com

Spring Hill Nurseries
110 West Elm St
Tipp City, OH 45371-1699
(513) 354-1509
springhillnursery.com

White Flower Farm
P.O. Box 50
Litchfield, CT 06759-0050
(800) 503-9624
whiteflowerfarm.com

SEED CATALOGUES

Baker Creek Heirloom Seeds
2278 Baker Creek Rd
Mansfield, MO 65704
(417) 924-8917
rareseeds.com

W. Atlee Burpee Co.
300 Park Ave, Warminster, PA 18974
(215) 674-4900
burpee.com

RESOURCES

The Cook's Garden
P.O. Box C5030
Warminster, PA 18974-0574
(800) 457-9703
cooksgarden.com

Gurney's Seed & Nursery Co.
P.O. Box 4178
Greendale, IN 47025-4178
(812) 260-2153
gurneys.com

Johnny's Selected Seeds
955 Benton Avenue
Winslow, Maine 04901
(877) 564-6697
johnnyseeds.com

Park Seed Co.
3507 Cokesbury Road
Hodges, SC 29653
(800) 845-3369
parkseed.com

Peaceful Valley Farm Supply
PO Box 2209, 125 Clydesdale Court
Grass Valley, CA 95945
(888) 784-1722
groworganic.com

Seed Savers Exchange
3094 North Winn Rd
Decorah, Iowa 52101
(563) 382-5990
seedsavers.org

Territorial Seed Company
PO Box 158
Cottage Grove, OR 97424
(800) 626-0866
territorialseed.com

Tomato Growers Supply Co.
P.O. Box 60015
Fort Myers, FL 33906
(888) 478-7333
tomatogrowers.com

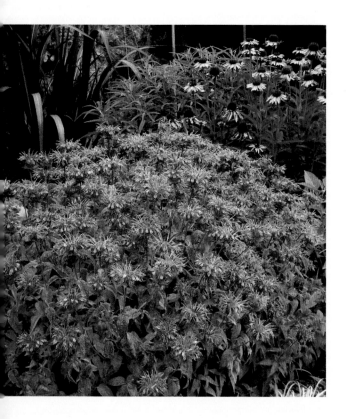

ACKNOWLEDGMENTS

It will come as a shock to no one that it takes a lot of people to pull off a book about gardening, cancer, nutrition and spirituality, so my apologies ahead of time for my acknowledgments appearing like an Academy Awards acceptance speech. The older I get, the more convinced I am that we were meant to live in community and to help one another out, and I call my community my Tribe. So here is my Tribe, for whom I am profoundly grateful:

My St. Lynn's Press family – because you are like family. Paul, Cathy, Holly, Chloe – you all take my meanderings and stream of consciousness tomfoolery and turn it into something way cooler than anything I could have created on my own. You knew this book could be more than what I had originally envisioned it to be, and for that, I am deeply grateful.

To Bill Bastas, Gayle Wismar, Nathan Wells, Deborah Carroll, Julia Campbell, Rick Bickling, Mimi San Pedro, Fred Hartwig, Chris Overbeek, Scooter Sanders, Donna Mercer, Lisa McVey, Patti Waldrup, Marisol Avila, Ruby Cortez, Rebecca Sweet, Olivia Moreno and Howard Davis – I give thanks for you and your willingness to share your stories of survivorship within these pages. Whether it was participating in a Saturday photo shoot, sending images of you in your garden, or appearing in a Survivor Spotlight, you gave us a peek into your world in an effort to help other Survivors. Angel wings for you all.

To Joe Lamp'l, Steve Bender, Fran Sorin, Ray Anne Evans, Naomi Sachs, Andie Redwine, Shirley Bovshow, Dr. Robin Mayfield, Dr. Carlos Rubin de Celis, Jacqueline Jensen, LaManda Joy Minikel, Rebecca Sweet, Linda Lehmusvirta, Susan Gonzalez, Denise Mickelsen, Kylee Baumle, Pam Penick, Chris McLaughlin, Nancy Ondra and Florence Strang – many, many thanks for lending your professional endorsements of this book to get it into the hands of those who can benefit from it. Your confidence in me and of this project will never be forgotten.

Some of the people I want to thank occupy more than one category of my gratitude, and their names appear more

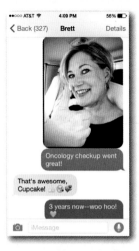

than once in these acknowledgments.

To my medical team – Dr. Carlos Rubin de Celis, Dr. Robin Mayfield, Jackie Jensen, Rhonda Bentura, Ellen Buentello and Sandra Enright – you all have supported me medically, emotionally, spiritually and physically. There are no words to thank you enough. In my tradition, there is a "valley of the shadow of death," and each of you has shown a strong and loving light as you walked with me from that valley into health again.

To Elissa Marie, who took time on a Sunday morning to help me with the cover photography of this book, and to Jen Neve, who guided me with information about good soil bacteria — thank you. And thanks to Su Reid-St. John from Bonnie Plants who took her own time to find plant images for me — it's truly appreciated! Friends like you, who know things I don't, and are readily willing to share your knowledge and time, are priceless.

To my forever friends Kylee Baumle, Rebecca Sweet, Theresa Loe, Laura

Livengood, Susan Morrison, Helen Weis, Sherry Richardson, Jacque Gregory, Terri Curtis, Paul Fafard, Todd Zivin, Robin Mayfield, and DGS (you know who you are), I love you all like family. If I could get a tattoo with all of your names on it, I would. Well, I probably wouldn't, but I still love each one of you dearly. Your support and encouragement of me goes way beyond the expectation of normal friendship.

To my family – Phil & Turid, Celia & Bro, Claire & Al, Laura & Mike, Carl & Kristi, Wendy & Dave, Norma and my fabulous nieces and nephews – you are my rock. I know family is expected to show up and say cheers, but many don't. You did. And do. You all are the greatest blessings in my life.

And to the three most important men in my life: Brett, Max and Luke – you give me three of the best reasons every single day to get up, show up, give thanks and keep moving forward. Each of you is woven into my heart in a way that can never be fully understood or expressed. I love you.

And for cancer survivors everywhere – each of you has your own journey, your own path, your own experiences and your own tribes to see you through. I hope this book helps you get to your place of hope, healing and joy.

Thank you all for being in my Tribe. ∿

ABOUT THE AUTHOR

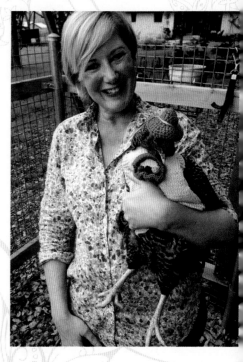

Jenny Peterson is a landscape designer, writer, speaker and breast cancer survivor who comes from a family of gardeners and creators. She enjoys helping her design clients, readers and students create garden spaces that enrich and improve the quality of their lives, from xeriscapes and small spaces to indoor gardens and meditation areas.

She has written for a number of home, garden and lifestyle publications and sites, including *Austin Home, Fine Gardening, Oklahoma Gardener* and *Houzz,* and has been a brand ambassador for the Proven Winners plant brand and Sanctuary Soil. She speaks to garden clubs and flower and garden shows around the country, and has recently teamed with Craftsy.com to create and instruct a video class, "Gorgeous Garden Design: Function & Style."

Her first book, *Indoor Plant Décor: The Design Stylebook for Houseplants* (St. Lynn's Press 2013) was co-authored with Kylee Baumle, and was named one of the Top 20 on Amazon in its category for 2013.

And because Jenny believes that everyone should have a little-known fact to share about themselves, she confides that she and the members of her high school marching band were extras in a Jackie Chan martial arts movie in the 1980s. She lives, works and gardens on a full acre in Austin, Texas, where she has chickens, goats and ducks. She has two sons, Max and Luke, who are her life's greatest creations, and her fiancé Brett who cheerfully digs holes where she points. ❧

INDEX

INDEX

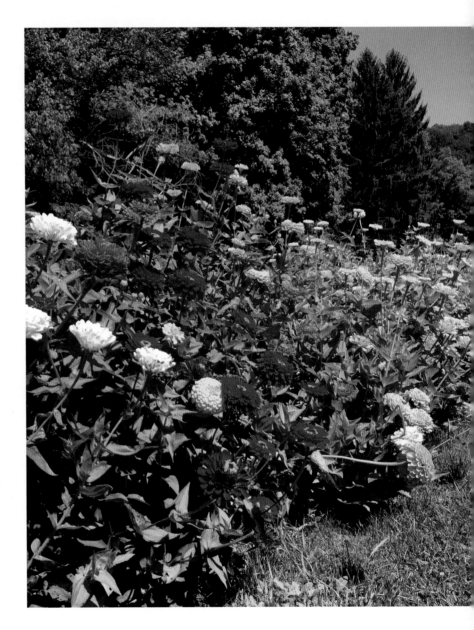

OTHER BOOKS FROM ST. LYNN'S PRESS

www.stlynnspress.com

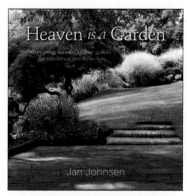

Heaven is a Garden
by Jan Johnsen
160 pages • Hardback • ISBN: 978-0-9855622-9-8

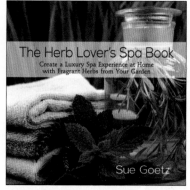

The Herb Lover's Spa Book
by Sue Goetz
192 pages • Hardback • ISBN: 978-0-9892688-6-8

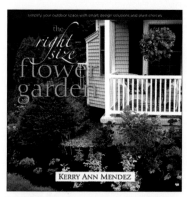

The Right-Size Flower Garden
by Kerry Mendez
160 pages • Hardback • ISBN: 978-0-9892688-7-5

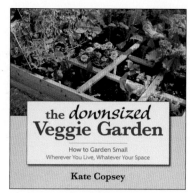

The Downsized Veggie Garden
by Kate Copsey
160 pages • Hardback • ISBN: 978-1-943366-00-2